BACK SMART

DANIEL KASSICIEH, D.O., FAAN

BOARD CERTIFIED NEUROLOGIST

FELLOW AMERICAN ACADEMY OF NEUROLOGY

Published By:

Suncoast Digital Press
Sarasota, Florida

www.suncoastdigitalpress.com

Printed in the United States of America

ISBN 978-1-939237-11-8

FIRST EDITION

DEDICATION

This book is dedicated to my patients and all those who suffer from back and neck pain.

I wrote this book to give you all hope that there is an answer to your pain and suffering that does not involve surgery or narcotics. The answer to a better quality of life is only a few pages away.

CONTENTS

PREFACE

Picture a directory sign, the kind you see in a building on the wall near an elevator which lists the suite occupant names and location. On this directory, one nameplate reads: CONSERVATIVE TREATMENT AND NATURAL HEALING, Suite 201. Another nameplate: SURGICAL SPINE ASSOCIATES, Suite 220. Which office do you want to visit first?

Unfortunately, most people do not realize that they have this **choice** when they are suffering with terrible neck or back pain. In fact, in many cases, their Board-Certified medical doctor whom they trust has advised them they have no choice but to go see a spine surgeon. They are told that surgery is their only option. But you DO have a choice and I work with patients every day who I ensure are enlightened and empowered to make smart decisions about their neck and back pain treatment—and you can, too.

I am so passionate about educating people to the facts that I spend most of my weekends teaching, speaking, and now, writing this book. My teachings include these basics:

- Low back pain is second only to the common cold as a cause of lost days at work. It is also one of the most common reasons to visit a doctor's office or a hospital's emergency department. It is the second most common neurologic complaint in the United States, second only to headache.

- For most people, even those with nerve root irritation (sciatica), their symptoms will improve within two months no matter what treatment is used, even if no treatment is given – Natural Healing.

- Doctors usually refer to back pain as acute if it has been present for less than a 6 weeks and chronic if it lasts for a longer than three months.

- For the majority (97%) of neck and back pain sufferers– surgery is not, and will never be, the answer.

One day, as I was showing some illustrations to a patient in order to help her understand exactly why surgery, in her case, was not going to help with her lower back pain, she asked me, "How in the world was I supposed to know this?" Well, in the next several chapters, you will be clued in and shown everything you need to learn in order to understand your very real options, many of which no doctor has revealed to you before.

Each CASE STUDY that I have included is a true story, with the patient's name changed for privacy. Let's look at seven crucial reasons to avoid spine surgery and explore other solutions.

INTRODUCTION

A Life Destroyed by Unnecessary Back Surgery

(How Not to Manage Lower Back Pain)

This is an actual case of an individual who had a simple low back muscle strain. Through alarming (but all too common) medical mismanagement, he became completely disabled.

Can you recall a time when you lifted a heavy box or moved a couch and ended up with back and/or neck pain? It's very common. This example well-illustrates how a back muscle strain injury can easily be misdiagnosed and mismanaged, essentially ruining your life. I am sharing this case study here as it demonstrates how easily you can be led down the wrong path, to your own demise. The point is, this could have been anyone. All names and specific details have been changed to maintain privacy.

CASE STUDY

"Jack" was a forty-eight year old male who had a twisting back strain injury. He had some lower back pain following this non-traumatic back strain. His neurological exam was normal and did not show any evidence of nerve root or "spinal" involvement. He continued working but his back pain worsened. He first saw an orthopedic surgeon one month after the injury.

The orthopedic surgeon (who was not a spine surgeon) *correctly diagnosed* back strain injury. The doctor gave him non-narcotic medications and Jack gradually improved. Approximately five months later, he had a flare up of his back pain. Also, he was having some vague pain in the right leg, but had a history of a "bad knee" on the right for 10 years prior to the back injury.

He had undergone knee surgery and wore a knee brace since the time of the knee surgery to the present.

The patient was complaining of right lower back pain (his original complaint) but now had some nonspecific *right* leg symptoms. Despite a normal neurological exam and no testing being performed, the orthopedic surgeon *incorrectly* concluded that the patient had a "hot right S1 disc problem." He sent the patient to a neurosurgeon. Keep in mind, this patient had chronic right knee pain and wore a brace.

In taking a history from Jack, the neurosurgeon noted that the patient had two prior right knee surgeries. During his exam, he found no weakness or sensory loss but did note the patient "had trouble standing on his tiptoes on the right." On this basis, the neurosurgeon concluded that the patient also had a right S1 disc problem. (I must note that patients with chronic knee pain after two knee surgeries *typically* have trouble standing on their toes, due to knee pain.)

An MRI of the lower back was ordered. This showed a mild right-sided disc protrusion at the L5-S1 level, but the radiologist who interpreted the MRI noted that the S1 nerve root was freely exiting below the *mild* disc protrusion. There was *no* nerve compression. The neurosurgeon proceeded to do right lower back surgery on Jack. After some rehabilitation, over several months, he was doing better. It should be noted that Jack never received any conservative therapy (the standard of care) prior to his back surgery. The rehabilitation that he got after surgery most likely would have cleared Jack's pain without him ever having surgery—conservative treatment is the first line, standard of care for treatment of all similar back pain cases.

Jack did well until one year later. He again had another flare up of his low back pain, but was now having complaints of *left* leg pain. The same neurosurgeon did a neurological exam and did not find any neurological abnormalities. Another MRI lumbar spine was ordered to "see if we are dealing with a left L4-5 or L5-S1 herniated disc."

Again, the neurosurgeon's exam did not show any findings of nerve root compression and no conservative therapy was ordered. This time, narcotics were prescribed. The lumbar spine MRI was performed and, according to the neurosurgeon's own words, the resulting image "was unremarkable." This means that even the neurosurgeon did not find anything on the study to explain Jack's new lower back or *left* leg pain. His original complaint, remember, was nonspecific *right* leg pain.

The neurosurgeon stated specifically that there was no disc herniation on either side of the spine. Physical therapy was ordered after the MRI test. Jack's pain persisted. Yet another lumbar spine MRI was ordered, only three months after the first. This third MRI, once again, did not show any clinically significant, surgically treatable findings. The third MRI study, read by a different radiologist, showed the same findings as the first. Epidural steroid injections were given for Jack's back pain but did not provide any relief.

Jack continued to have complaints of lower back pain with non-specific left leg complaints. He was seen by a rehabilitation physician, who also did not find any neurological problems to explain Jack's pain. An intensive course of rehabilitation was undertaken without significant improvement. Jack came under the care of another neurosurgeon. This new neurosurgeon again found no clinically significant findings on Jack's exam. On the basis of reading the three MRI reports mentioned above only, and without him personally reviewing the MRI films, this neurosurgeon recommended that Jack undergo a complex, left sided L4-L5 spine surgical procedure. Remember, all three MRI scans failed to show *anything* that would explain Jack's leg pains.

This surgery was performed and Jack did poorly, as one would expect. This exactly demonstrates that doing surgery based on the patient's complaints, lack of specific MRI abnormalities or findings on exam plus poor surgical judgment will ultimately result in a bad outcome. Jack was given the status of total permanent disability after the second back surgery. This is a classic case of a patient being made disabled by inappropriate, unnecessary spine surgery. This scenario, unfortunately, repeats itself thousands of times a year in the United States.

Fast forward to twenty years after the original muscle strain injury and Jack is still having back and bilateral leg pain complaints. **He has seen over 13 physicians.** His current treating physician is doing numerous injections monthly, using narcotics and other acute pain treatment medications, for a 20-year old problem! Injection therapy, of any kind, is not indicated for chronic lower back pain and post-laminectomy syndrome; particularly for a pain problem that arose 20 years ago.

Let's look at this case from the beginning. Jack's original treating physician, an orthopedic surgeon, concluded that just because he had right leg pain, it "had to be" due to a disc herniation. The fact of the matter is that the patient had been enduring chronic right leg pain from a knee injury that had occurred 10 years prior to his back injury.

The second mistake was when the first neurosurgeon concluded that an MRI finding was the cause of the patient's right leg pain—even when the radiologist reading the MRI scan stated in his report that the right S1 nerve root was not compromised. As reported in the *New England Journal of Medicine*,[1]

> "There is general agreement that patients with acute, nonspecific spine pain or nonlocalizable lumbosacral radiculopathy (without neurologic signs or significant neurologic symptoms) require only conservative medical management. Patients should abstain from heavy lifting or other activities that aggravate the pain. Bed rest is not helpful and has been shown to delay recovery."

Jack had no significant neurological symptoms or exam findings but the neurosurgeon operated on him anyway. You cannot surgically fix *normal*.

The third major medical error in this case was that of the second neurosurgeon. For his second back pain episode, Jack went to a neurosurgeon for help. Opposite from a year prior, now he had low back and LEFT leg pain-the leg which was originally without symptoms. Two MRI low back scans were performed and did not show any clinically, or surgically, significant findings. Jack's first neurosurgeon had pointed that out.

Jack's second neurosurgeon, only after reading the two MRI reports, concluded that "the patient needed immediate surgery." He also said that no conservative treatment should be utilized prior to surgery. A double jeopardy here. First, he did not treat the patient conservatively for a minimum of eight weeks. Second, which is *inexcusable*, he recommended a complex spine surgery on the basis of reading the reports only, not reviewing the MRI scans himself and correlating them with the patient's neurological exam.

Reported in the *Annals of Internal Medicine*: "Diagnostic imaging of the spine has a high rate of abnormal findings in asymptomatic persons. In studies of lumbar spine MRI evaluation in *asymptomatic* adults, herniated disks were found in 9-76% of patients, bulging disks in 20-81%, degenerative disks in 46-93% and annular tears in 14-56%. Therefore, MRI imaging should be used in carefully selected patients and interpreted with appropriate clinical correlation.[2,3]

Following his second back surgery, Jack had to go on total, **permanent disability**. Here is a man whose entire life was forever damaged by unnecessary back surgery. This is a true story and **could happen just as easily to you**. Beware of any spine surgeon who is quick to recommend back or neck surgery without a full course of conservative management. The natural course of back and neck pain is to improve on its own over six to eight weeks with conservative treatment. Take your MRI scan and get another opinion.

> Neck and back pain usually have nothing to do with the spine or spinal nerves.

Unfortunately, Jack then received even more abuse. His treating physician prescribed several medications that have no place in managing chronic low back pain. Additionally, he was injecting Jack's back every month with local anesthetics, basically masking pain for a few hours with novocaine. The effectiveness of selective nerve root blocks at the lumbosacral levels has been studied and determined to be ineffective. A further concern is that a placebo response rate of 38% was reported.[4]

Trigger point injections are not indicated for nonspecific acute or chronic low back pain, and sacroiliac joint injections are not indicated in the routine management of low back pain.[5] A trigger point injection is nothing more that injecting novocaine into various tender spots along a muscle or group of muscles. This has been shown to have virtually no lasting pain relief and certainly will not treat the underlying condition.

Myofascial pain syndrome is a common localized musculoskeletal pain syndrome caused by myofascial trigger points located at muscle, fascia, or tendinous insertions, affecting up to 95% of people with chronic pain disorders. Repeated trigger point injections should be avoided, and corticosteroids should not be injected into trigger points.[6] Again, we need to look for the underlying cause of this muscle pain. Most commonly, we see muscle weakness, shortened muscle length ("tightness"), and loss of flexibility. All of these underlying causes of pain need to be corrected to have effective, lasting pain relief.

CHAPTER 1

Back Pain Will Clear on Its Own
or Heal with Conservative Treatment

Our bodies are designed to automatically work to self-repair and heal, and they do this 24/7, even when we are asleep. This natural healing is such an effective process that we often are unaware that there were actually problems existing which needed attention. Other times, we can witness the process of our body fixing a serious issue, all without the help of medicine or medical treatment, and may view it as nothing short of miraculous. For example, a broken bone prompts the body to start growing new bone cells, in the precisely right location only, and then hardens and fuses them to existing bone. With time, the fracture disappears. The same thing happens in most cases of back problems—the causes of the pain heal and clear up on their own, or with conservative therapy.

Natural Treatment Methods—Best Choices

For many people, taking an anti-inflammatory non-prescription medication such as aspirin, ibuprofen, or naproxen can provide relief. Using an ice pack wrapped in a light towel, applied to your back for 20 minutes, 2-3 times daily, can relieve pain and reduce inflammation in the injured area. (It is best to avoid heat in situations of acute back or neck strain.) The point is, temporary relief of symptomatic pain is all that you may need while your body is working to resolve the issue which is causing the pain.

For cases of pain that last for more than a few days, acupuncture and/or massage therapy is frequently beneficial. Simply relaxing the muscles often reduces pain significantly. If your pain continues, visit your physician and get a referral for physical therapy and/or osteopathic manipulation therapy.

It is important that if you have lower back pain, start and continue doing back exercises regularly to maintain a more healthy back and avoid future attacks of back pain. Long ago, "bed rest" may have been prescribed for back pain, but now we know that stretching and exercise are better, by far, for relief and good back conditioning. Our bodies are designed for movement, and more movement equals more overall health.

Pain may be partly caused by weak abdominal muscles. Since your abs are the front anchor of your spine, if they are weak, then the other structures supporting your spine (your back muscles, for example) will have to work harder. By developing stronger core muscles, you'll be less likely to injure or strain your back muscles.

Back pain is often uncomfortable and activity-limiting without being debilitating. That is, you may not be able to lift your child, jog around the block, or wear high-heeled shoes as you usually would be able to do, but you can get out of bed, dress, and walk, even though your back is hurting. The treatment of these minimally-limiting conditions should be simple home remedies as previously mentioned. If your pain continues or worsens, a visit to a back pain specialist—who is not a surgeon—would be appropriate. A detailed history and physical exam will be performed, followed by a prescribed course of conservative therapy.

Please note that at no point has neuroimaging (MRI scanning) been mentioned in the routine assessment and treatment of neck or lower back pain, as it is not medically necessary. As one journal notes:

"…In patients with non-specific acute low back pain, without the red flags, a conservative approach is preferable, with assessment in 4–6 weeks. The natural history of low back pain is favorable with improvement over time… There is limited role of imaging in non-specific acute low back pain without the red flags, as the findings correlate poorly with symptoms."[7]

Conservative therapy is the treatment of choice for almost every case of neck or back pain. Of course, that is when no serious underlying disease (which is exceedingly rare) is suspected. Narcotic medications should be avoided in most cases. Painkillers only mask the pain and do nothing to clear the causes of pain, while contributing to potential over-use, serious addiction and even death. Patients generally feel poorly when taking pain medications with little, if any, lasting relief.

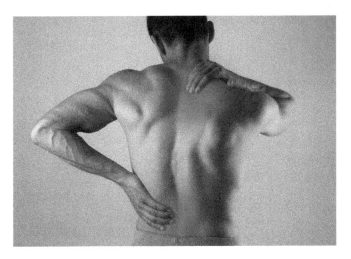

Neck and back pain frequently occur together.

Prescription painkillers are habit-forming, addictive, and fall into the category of "controlled substances." Controlled substances are medications that can cause physical and mental dependence, and the manufacturing, possession, and use of these medications is regulated by law. How controlled substances are regulated and classified by the Drug Enforcement Administration (DEA) is based on how likely they are to cause dependence. An example of a controlled substance includes hydrocodone, one of many opioid pain medications and one of the most overused. Opioid addiction has become a major health concern and cause of death in the United States. The Center for Disease Control (CDC) reports that approximately 70,000 Americans die from narcotic overdose annually.

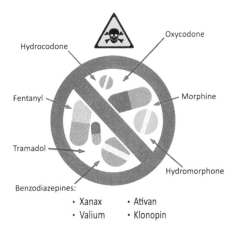

Avoid narcotic treatment for neck or back pain.

3

There is no such imagined person you could label as a "typical" drug addict. All too many individuals of all ages and backgrounds with lower back pain have become "accidental" addicts due to taking powerful painkillers (e.g., hydrocodone, oxycodone, Oxycontin). These dangerously addictive drugs are not needed to successfully treat and manage neck and back pain. Narcotics cure nothing. They can mask the painful symptoms while the body is healing itself, but because of their addictive traits, patients continue the use beyond the symptom-relief period. This leads to serious health problems and sometimes death. Conservative, non-invasive, non-narcotic therapy is the treatment of choice in over 95% of routine cases of back and neck pain.

The Most Effective Therapies for Lower Back Pain

Physical Therapy

The type of physical therapy that you get is important. Routine physical therapy consisting of ultrasound, electrical stimulation, and hot/cold packs makes little or no difference and is not productive. Effective physical therapy consists of hands-on manual physical therapy to help relax and stretch the muscles which are in painful spasm, and to correct any joint mobility problems. This is then followed with proper muscle stretching, strengthening, and conditioning. Healthy, conditioned back and abdominal muscles avoid future back and neck pain issues.

Osteopathic Manipulative Therapy (OMT) and Chiropractic

Osteopathic manipulative therapy (OMT) is a well-known hands-on treatment. Multiple published studies have shown proven benefits of OMT in the conservative management of neck and back pain.[8]

Many people find that chiropractic treatment helps to relieve back pain, sometimes almost instantly. Chiropractors use various hands-on spinal manipulation and other treatments, the theory being that proper alignment of the body's musculoskeletal structure, particularly the spine, will enable the body to heal itself without surgery or medication. Manipulation is used to restore mobility to joints restricted by tissue injury caused by a traumatic event, such as falling, or repetitive stress, such as sitting without proper back support.

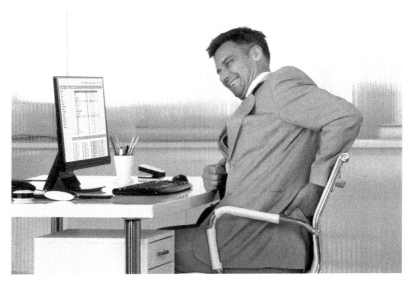

And about your joints—a foot, ankle, knee, hip, sacroiliac or tailbone joint mobility problems can cause or aggravate back pain. Hip joint problems and unequal leg length commonly cause back and leg pain, these symptoms having nothing to do with the spine. It is absolutely necessary that your treatment therapist address these areas to ensure proper joint mobility.

Acupuncture for Back Pain

Acupuncture is a 2,500-year-old therapy that has been proven in many countries to be a safe, effective treatment for back pain. One peer-reviewed study in a respected Western medical journal reported the following:

"Lower back pain improved after acupuncture treatment for at least six months. Effectiveness of acupuncture …was almost twice that of conventional therapy."[9]

Gua sha Massage

Sometimes patients may continue to experience neck and back pain even after having surgery, taking drugs, or receiving osteopathic manipulation, acupuncture, and/or massage.

> Most causes of neck and back pain have nothing to do with the spine or spinal nerves.

These patients often suffer from pain that does not have an identifiable cause. However, most neck and back pain comes from disorders of the soft tissue, having nothing to do with the spine or spinal nerves.

Gua Sha Scraping Tool

Normal Sha Response

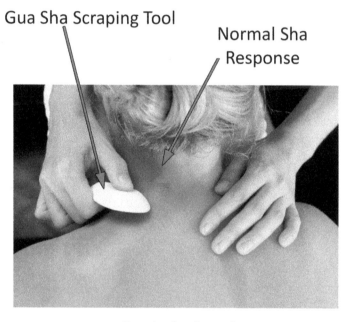

Gua sha for the neck

There is a simple acupuncture-related Chinese massage technique known as *gua sha,* and it clearly is one of the most effective therapies for neck or back pain stemming from soft tissue disorders.

Gua sha can help eliminate the accumulated toxins in the soft tissue. *Gua sha* also increases fresh, oxygenated blood flow to the inflamed tissue, aiding further in healing. It involves putting pressure on the skin with a massage tool. Redness with a bruised look ("sha") is normal to treated areas. This is painless and indicates a good therapeutic response.

Best of all, *gua sha* serves as a simple, non-invasive pain relieving therapy.

The Truth About Massage

Conclusions of four peer-reviewed research studies which affirm the efficacy of massage in the treatment of lower back pain are listed below.

1. People with subacute low back pain were put into four groups. The groups were comprehensive massage therapy, soft tissue manipulation only, exercise with posture education, and a placebo group with a sham laser therapy. After 1 month, 63% of the comprehensive massage therapy group reported no pain, compared to 27% of the soft tissue manipulation group, 14% of the exercise group and 0% of the placebo group.[10]

2. Two hundred sixty-two (262) patients aged 20 to 70 years with persistent back pain were to receive Traditional Chinese Medical acupuncture, therapeutic massage, or self-care educational materials for the 10-week study. Conclusions were that massage was superior to self-care on the symptom scale. Massage was also superior to acupuncture. After one year, massage was not better than self-care, but proved better than acupuncture. The massage group used the least medications and had the lowest costs of subsequent care.[11]

3. A randomized study of chiropractic, massage, corset and transcutaneous muscle stimulation (TMS) was conducted in patients with low back pain. Patients were enrolled for a period of three weeks and were evaluated once a week by questionnaires, visual analog scale, range of motion, maximum voluntary extension effort, straight leg raising and a fatigue test. After three weeks, the chiropractic group scored the greatest improvements in flexion and pain while the massage group had the best extension effort and fatigue time, and the TMS group the best extension.[12]

4. Four hundred (400) patients were randomly assigned to a structural massage group, relaxation massage group, or a usual care group. The usual care group included medications, physical therapy and back exercises. The structural massage group received neuromuscular and musculoskeletal massage and the relaxation massage was Swedish massage. Each massage participant received a one-hour massage, once a week, for 10 weeks. The patients were measured by amount of medications, symptoms, and ability to perform activities at 10 weeks, 6 months, and 1 year. Both massage groups showed significant increases in reduction of symptoms and daily functions. At 6 months, the massage groups still showed some improvement, but after one year all three groups were the same. This study shows that massage can be helpful in reducing back pain.[13]

Improvement is Often Independent of Treatment

The American College of Physicians concluded that most patients with acute or subacute low back pain will improve over time. This improvement occurred independent of treatment given. Treatment modalities included heat, massage, acupuncture or spinal manipulation. Pharmacological treatment recommendations were limited to anti-inflammatory agents and muscle relaxants. Of particular note was that steroid medications like cortisone and Prednisone were not particularly effective for pain relief.[14]

Oral steroids, either tablets or "dose-packs," have no beneficial effect on clearing the back or neck pain you are experiencing. Additionally, steroids have well known side effects such as elevated blood sugar, temporary worsening of diabetes, elevated blood pressure, severe insomnia, accelerated osteoporosis and spontaneous bone fractures. Steroids can also accelerate the development of cataracts.

In clinical studies, oral steroids have not been shown to be any more effective than placebos[15] and should be avoided in the treatment of neck and back pain. Treatment guidelines such as the AHRQ (see Appendix) specifically state that oral steroids are not indicated in the treatment of acute, subacute or chronic neck or back pain.

For chronic low back pain, ACP recommendations included primarily non-pharmacologic treatment with exercise (*tai chi*, yoga, stretching), acupuncture, stress reduction, cognitive behavioral therapy, and spinal manipulation. In those individuals who use these treatments and continue to have back pain, combination therapy with anti-inflammatory agents and second line therapies such as duloxetine or low-dose tramadol may be considered.

The summary of recommendations for your back pain includes patient education and reassurance that your acute or subacute low back pain will improve over time, with or without conservative therapies. Even your sciatica (leg pain) has a high likelihood for improvement over a four-week period. Remain as active as can be tolerated and try self-care options such as ice, stretching, and other non-invasive treatments. Keep everything out of your back pockets since sitting on anything means uneven pelvic pressure and your spine will tilt to one side. This puts strain on the back and hip muscles and can significantly contribute to back and hip pain.

Since driving or riding in a car means sitting (sometimes for long distances), pay attention to your posture and car seat position. When traveling, allow for frequent stops; get out of the car and move around. It is also very helpful to put a towel roll in the seat of your car. Place it where the back of the seat meets the seat cushion. This provides back support that even the best car seats or other back support devices cannot do. It is also the least expensive, effective treatment to prevent back pain. Spine imaging and any type of invasive treatment (epidural steroids, radio frequency ablation, or surgery) do not even enter into therapeutic consideration.

The sacrum (tailbone) is a common cause of back and even leg pain. The sacrum is at the end of the spine and connects the two halves of the hip bones together, in conjunction with the end of the spine. The main movement of the sacrum is slight, but is basically forward or backward.

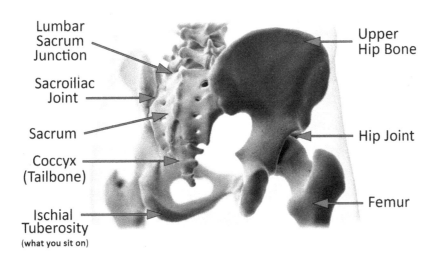

Sacrum articulating with pelvic bones

When you bend or extend your back, the sacrum will normally move the opposite direction. Sometimes, the sacrum gets "stuck" in rotation. When this happens, the normal motion of the lower back, spine, and sacrum becomes restricted, sometimes causing severe back pain. Since many muscles, tendons, and ligaments attach to the sacrum, don't underestimate its importance. (Tip: Reaching back to massage your tailbone area with your fist can often relieve pain in that and other areas of your back, immediately.)

To compensate for sacral misalignment, the back muscles tighten up and cause more pain. It is a vicious cycle that needs proper treatment to restore normal movement, thereby eliminating pain. This is where OMT, manual hands-on physical therapy, or acupuncture techniques can help. Proper mobility of the sacroiliac joint in conjunction with the lumbar spine is essential in maintaining good back mechanics and a pain-free state.

Pelvic Ligaments Front View

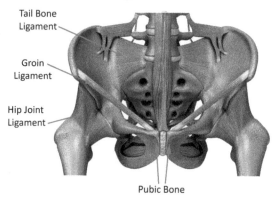

Pelvic Ligaments Rear View

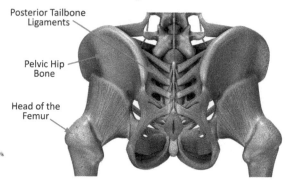

Ligaments attaching to sacrum and hip joints

In case of more persistent spasm or pain, acupuncture can also help. Topical analgesic creams applied to sore muscles may provide temporary benefits, as well. With one or more of these combined therapies, the vast majority (95%+) of cases of lower back or neck pain can be treated successfully. No invasive procedures such as epidural steroids, facet injections, or spine surgery are needed. MRI scanning specifically is not needed in the routine treatment and management of neck and back pain.

Doctor Recommendations to Consider

- Your doctor may offer one of these treatments: an exercise routine, a course of OMT, manual physical therapy including stretching and manipulation, or a course of acupuncture. If the treatment does not result in satisfactory improvement, adding another one of these may be suggested.

- Your doctor may put more emphasis on a structured exercise program, tailored to you, that may include core conditioning and other exercises to strengthen your lower back and abdominal muscles, as well as improve posture and flexibility. You will want to use proper form to avoid strain or injury, and your doctor may provide diagram instructions or recommend that your work with a skilled personal fitness trainer. The trainer will be familiar with active stretching and conditioning of affected muscles in your neck, shoulder, back and hips.

- Your doctor could recommend a course of manual therapy, including spinal manipulation, spinal mobilization, and massage. Treatment may be provided by a range of health professionals including an osteopathic physician, hands-on manual physiotherapist, chiropractor, or other health care professionals who have had specialized training in muscle and spine manual therapy.

- Acupuncture is often physician-recommended, and could include a course of treatments, up to a maximum of 10 sessions over a period of up to 12 weeks. Other types of acupuncture therapies, such as gua sha, may be indicated as well.

- Do not expect your doctor to offer X-rays, CT, or MRI of the lumbar spine for the management of non-specific low back pain. They could offer an MRI scan within the context of specific neurological deficit on examination or for an opinion on spinal surgery, but should do this only if indicated. The same is true for neck pain problems. Remember: The majority of cases of neck or back pain do not need MRI scanning or surgery.

- Most physicians will recommend that you do regular home exercises for neck and back pain. These are critical in acute pain relief as well as maintenance therapy to avoid future attacks. Self-care practices should also include practicing good posture and not sitting for prolonged periods. You will probably be advised to keep items out of your back pockets, as sitting on these can trigger or make back pain worse. Also, you should learn to keep a towel roll in your car seat, at all times, to provide extra back support that even the best car seats do not provide.

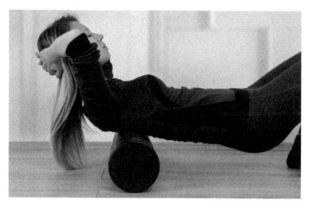

Foam roll to stretch out back, hip, and leg muscles

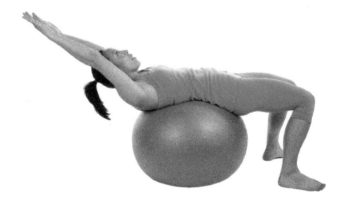

Using yoga ball for back stretching

- Best Conservative Therapy Choices
- Daily Neck and Back Exercises
- Physical Therapy
- Core Conditioning Training
- Weight Loss
- Osteopathic Manipulation Therapy
- Chiropractic
- Acupuncture and *gua sha*

- **Regular General Exercise**
  - Weight Training
  - Cardiovascular
  - Yoga and Stretching
  - Qualified Personal Trainer
- **Non-Narcotic Pain Medications**
  - Anti-inflammatory medication
  - Muscle relaxants
  - Topical analgesics
- **Massage Therapy**
- **Towel roll in car seat**
- **Stop Smoking**

Self-massage can also help. Massaging of the neck, upper arm, hip, buttocks and thigh muscles is relaxing and can provide pain relief. A newer type hand held massage unit has been developed and is quite effective. These massagers are generically known as "muscle massage guns" and are an excellent way to direct focused, deep massage on specific, tight, aching muscles. You can use this at any time, basically on any sore, tight, aching muscle in your neck, back, hip, arm or legs.

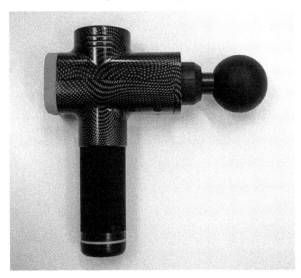

A muscle massage gun can become your favorite pain relief tool

There are many muscles involved in your pelvic girdle, hips, and lower back. Any of these can be strained, causing pain.

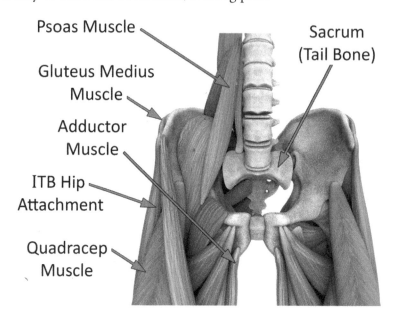

Psoas Muscle

Gluteus Medius Muscle

Adductor Muscle

ITB Hip Attachment

Quadracep Muscle

Sacrum (Tail Bone)

Complex frontal muscles of the back, hips and pelvis

"The best doctors give the least medicine."

—Benjamin Franklin

CHAPTER 2

Back Surgery–A Point of No Return

Once it's done, it's done. Back or neck surgery makes changes to your spine and surrounding structures which are permanent and not reversible.

A commitment to having spinal surgery on your neck or back, whether for the right or wrong reasons, is a one-way path. Once the surgeon makes the first incision and operates on your spine, the skeletal and spinal anatomy is forever changed. Your spine will never be the same—even if the surgery is successful.

> The first operation on a spine changes the skeletal and spinal anatomy permanently.

Spine surgery is never simple. Your spine is composed of many different structures that are changed with surgery. Let's look at the anatomy a moment: the spine is bone, held together by ligaments, with many muscles attaching to the bones by tendons. Many nerves are coming in and going out of the spinal cord and can be injured during spinal surgery.

Surgery Can Hurt More Than it Helps

In many back surgeries, part of the bone in the spine is removed, causing extra stress on the remaining spine. This usually results in a new source of pain and accelerated arthritis, in addition to scarring around the spine. In view of this, even with successful back surgery, the changes and new stresses put on your spine, above and below the original site of surgery, can result in additional pain. Unfortunately, this is often incorrectly perceived as an indication for additional back surgery.

Ligaments in the pelvis and lower lumbar spine change with age and these compound the problem. The younger you are when you have your first spine surgery, the greater the need for additional conservative treatment to avoid unnecessary surgery at a later date. If your pain is not completely relieved after surgery and beyond, and you again visit a spine surgeon, there is a high probability that you will be told that another surgery is needed. Beware of a white-lab-coat-wearing "surgical expert" holding a scalpel.

Giving the benefit of doubt that a back surgeon's motives are to help you solve your back pain, if all they know are surgery options, that's all that you will be told.

> ## Get a second opinion,
> ## preferably from a non-surgical physician.

Unfortunately, favorable outcomes in spine surgeries are in the minority. Over 500,000 back surgeries are done annually in the United States. Of these, half of all patients undergoing back surgery will not get the pain relief or desired results they had expected. One out of ten of these patients will have a permanently reduced quality of life and functionality following surgery. Permanently. Forever. A surgical procedure on your spine is a non-reversible process. Successful or more commonly not, the damage has been done.

Am I making my point too vigorously? With a back surgery failure rate of over 50%, don't you agree that you should always reconsider whether it is the proper choice of treatment? Get a second opinion, preferably from a non-surgical physician—a neurologist or physical medicine specialist familiar with conservative neck and back pain treatment. (If you go for another opinion from another surgeon, you will get another surgery-biased recommendation.)

The important fact to remember is that less than 1 out of 100 patients with back pain ever actually require surgery. The same is true for neck pain. Even in cases of a herniated disc, history shows that that these will usually heal with conservative therapies in 4 to 8 weeks. Your MRI showing "herniated disc(s)" does not mean that any of these are causing you any pain, numbness or require surgical treatment.

Every day I see patients who are shocked to learn that having a bulging or herniated disc does not equal having neck or back pain…and that surgery is NOT the answer.

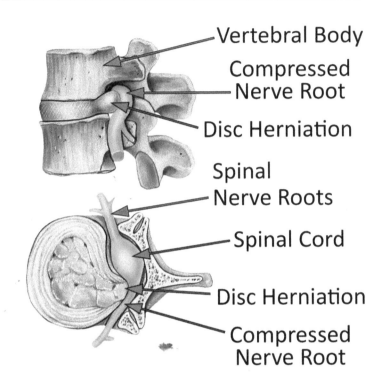

Left lateral disc herniation—compressing nerve root

As the Mayo Clinic (mayoclinic.org) explains: "A herniated disc refers to a problem with one of the rubbery cushions (discs) between the individual bones (vertebrae) that stack up to make your spine.

A spinal disc is a little like a jelly donut, with a softer center encased within a tougher exterior. Sometimes called a slipped disc or a ruptured disc, a herniated disc occurs when some of the softer 'jelly' pushes out through a tear in the tougher exterior.

A herniated disc can irritate nearby nerves and result in pain, numbness or weakness in an arm or leg. On the other hand, many people experience no symptoms from a herniated disc. Most people who have a herniated disc(s) don't need surgery to correct the problem.

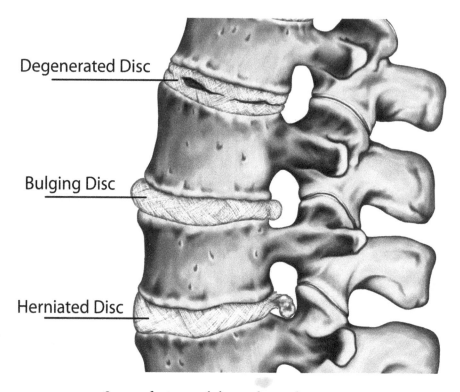

Degenerated Disc

Bulging Disc

Herniated Disc

Stages of spine and disc arthritic degeneration

Spine Institutes—A Profitable Business for Big Medicine

Spine institutes are popping up all over the United States. Their commercials and advertisements "inform" you, the consumer, that neck or back pain is somehow due to an abnormality of the spine such as "disc bulging, protrusions, tears and even disc herniations." It is inferred in these advertising campaigns that the abnormality seen on MRI scanning is responsible for the pain and that pain can be cured with spine surgery. Nothing could be further from the truth. Besides being unnecessary in most cases, remember, half of all back surgeries fail.

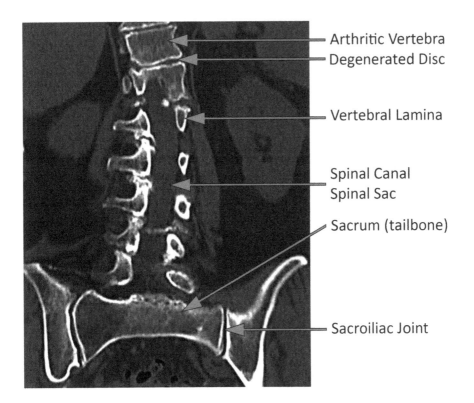

Arthritic Vertebra
Degenerated Disc

Vertebral Lamina

Spinal Canal
Spinal Sac

Sacrum (tailbone)

Sacroiliac Joint

CT scan arthritic spine degeneration changes—no stenosis

Many "Spine Institutes" advertise that if you suffer from chronic lower back pain, they have a "special, patented procedure" that will cure your pain. False! By definition, chronic low back pain has no identifiable cause or surgically treatable abnormality. A patented spine surgery procedure is not the magical cure for your chronic neck or back pain. At the end of the day, it is just another version of spine surgery.

What you should take note of is that all of these "special spine procedures" have in common one thing—*spine surgery.* The central theme of all "Spine Treatment" Centers is spine surgery, though this is not made clear in the massive advertising campaigns presented to the public. Frequently, the first consultation is "free." Free means they will have you come in with your MRI scan of the neck or lower back to meet briefly with someone. The study is read by one of their staff physicians, presumably a radiologist, although there are reports of chiropractors or other non-medical personnel looking at MRI scans to make the determination of surgical need—without you even having a detailed neurological exam!

Solely based on a generic medical staff member interpreting an MRI scan, the prospective patient (victim) will be told if he is a "candidate" for spine surgery. On that first visit, you may not even see a medical physician or have a complete neurological exam. If you do see a doctor, it will most likely be a surgeon explaining to you about what surgery it is that you are going to have, ***based on your MRI findings*** alone.

> ## MRI scans do not typically show the cause of neck or back pain.

Remember, 7 out of 10 people with no neck, back, arm or leg pain at all will have *abnormal* MRI findings, including disc herniations.[16,17,18] The "evidence" is shown to the patient who, understandably, is persuaded to think that the "abnormal" findings must be the problem. A detailed neurological and musculoskeletal exam should, of course, be performed in order to determine the actual cause of neck or back pain. Unfortunately this does not commonly occur. The "need for surgery" is frequently determined on the basis of MRI scan findings. Fact: MRI scans most commonly do not show the cause of neck or back pain and any changes on your MRI scanning typically do not explain your pain. Abnormalities on MRI spine scanning are common and usually do not show the cause of pain.[19,20]

Profit Seekers in Healers' Robes?

Spine treatment centers specializing in back pain are really just surgical centers disguised as healing centers. Conservative neck or back pain management and wellness are not their goal, but rather to ultimately perform spine surgery on you, necessary or not. Coincidentally, surgery pays big and pays well. Drive by your local "Spine Surgery Center" and ask yourself how they can afford that beautiful, multistory building.

Or, as in an event here in Florida, you might wonder why the striking, large building has an empty parking lot. The Laser Spine Institute, a "renowned spine center", closed suddenly, with no notice, leaving in the lurch hundreds of patients who had paid deposits. The *Tampa Bay Times* (March 1, 2019) reported: "Laser Spine notified its more than 500 employees on Friday that it would cease operations. Court losses may have played a role." Lawsuits too many to count!

We will be looking, later in this book, at what conditions need spine surgery and, mostly, at what does not. Beware: if what a "Spine Institute" tells you seems too good to be true, it almost always is. Do not be fooled by their reported "numbers of successful spine surgeries." **Their definition of "successful" may just be that the patient did not die**, certainly not whether or not the neck or back pain improved or cleared, or if the patient is no longer on chronic narcotics for pain management.

One national center promoting laser spine surgery claims a 96% success rate. Even the best neurosurgical spine centers do not have this high of success rate. *The overall national statistics for successful back surgery are less than 50%, with true success defined as pain free and no major, residual neurological problems.*

From *Bloomberg News*:

Unnecessary surgeries cost at least $150 billion a year, according to John Birkmeyer, director of the Center for Healthcare Outcomes & Policy at the University of Michigan. 'It's amazing how much evidence there is that fusions don't work, yet surgeons do them anyway,' said Sohail Mirza, a spine surgeon who chairs the Department of Orthopedics at Dartmouth Medical School in Hanover, New Hampshire. 'The only one who isn't benefitting from the equation is the patient...'[21]

Lasers are Just Another Way to Cut Your Body

A word on *laser* spine surgery: with any neck or back surgery, an incision needs to be made through the skin and subcutaneous tissue down to the spine. Whether a scalpel or laser is used, there is still an incision.

There are three major spinal surgical procedures performed: discectomies, foraminotomies and laminectomies. In any of these procedures, substituting a laser for a scalpel does not make any difference in what is done to you—it is the same procedure. Additionally, the reoperation rate for laser spine surgery is actually higher than traditional surgery.[22]

> The reoperation rate for laser spine surgery is higher than traditional surgery.

Is Spine Surgery a "Fast-Growing Business Opportunity"?

In the spine surgical industry, one "spine expert" projects a major growth over the next decade in the number of spine surgeries performed. The reasons they cite to justify more spine surgery include the following:

1. Increased activity: "more children and teens are playing sports than in years past... medical experts project significant growth in the spine care market."

2. Obesity: The US "is seeing higher rates of obesity now more than ever. Obesity stresses the spine leading to degeneration and spinal problems, which are projected to spur spinal [surgery] in the coming years."

3. Aging population: As the baby boomers are living into their 70s and 80s, "we can expect an influx of spinal problems...the aging population is expected to fuel the spinal [surgery] market over the next few years.

4. Better and smaller [surgical] techniques: "The spine care market is set to grow in the coming years... because we're getting better at performing operations. Patients who may have put off surgery are now willing to undergo [a spinal] operation because success rates have gotten better."

5. Better implants: "The spine [surgery] market will continue to thrive in the coming years because device manufacturers are getting better at developing more durable and biocompatible implants... This leads people who wouldn't normally undergo an operation to seek out surgical options because we're getting better at providing long term relief."[23]

There are a number of reasons that this reasoning is completely flawed. Of the five major points, the first two are contradictory. If it is true that children and teens are playing more sports, obesity would not be the growing problem that it is. Clearly, obesity is at epidemic levels in the United States.[24]

The third reason of an "aging population" is another incorrect justification for the increasing need for more spine surgery. Nothing could be further from the truth. If an aging population were a cause for more spine surgery, we would have already seen an exponential growth in the need for justified spine surgery due to people already living longer. Surgically treatable spinal disease should be on the basis of the patient's complaints, detailed neurologic exam and correlation with MRI findings. Remember, most cases of neck and back pain (97%) do not require surgical intervention. The remaining erroneous points make an assertion that advances in medical technology guarantee more successful outcomes, which is not true.

Sciatica – Not Always a Surgical Problem

Sciatica usually refers to pain beginning in the lower back and buttocks, radiating down the back of the leg. It most commonly affects only one leg. In common usage however, patients refer to any leg pains as "sciatica." Taken in this context, there are many causes of leg pain that have nothing to do with the spine or spinal nerves. Examples of this are hip arthritis, knee problems, iliotibial band syndrome, hamstring sprain, short leg syndrome, piriformis syndrome—just to name a few.

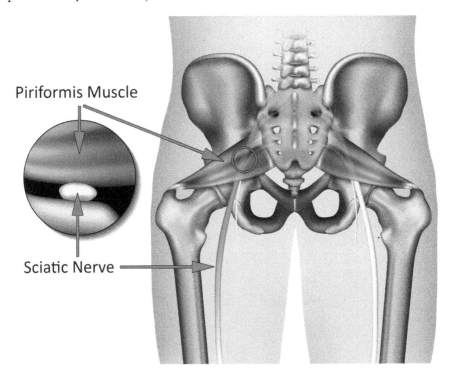

Piriformis Muscle

Sciatic Nerve

Sciatic nerve originating from base of spine, extending down back of leg

CASE STUDY

Iliotibial Band Syndrome—a different cause for leg pain

"Anne" is a 75-year-old patient with back and left leg pain. She was seen by an orthopedic spine surgeon who ordered an MRI lumbar spine scan. Her report showed some non-specific arthritic changes. Anne underwent spinal surgery to "fix" her back and leg pain. After surgery, she continued to have severe left leg pain which was worse than ever.

Seeing the same orthopedic surgeon again, she was found to have actually had a left hip fracture as a cause of her "sciatica." The fracture was completely missed prior to her back surgery. She needed surgical pinning of her hip fracture. This is a patient who underwent completely unnecessary back surgery. She continues to suffer from permanent back and leg pain to this day, due to Failed Back Surgery.

Leg pain is a common problem. We will all have leg pain at some time in our lives. Leg pain can be due to many causes including sciatic nerve pain, hip arthritis, knee injuries, leg muscle strains, or even foot problems. A common problem which can mimic sciatica pain is a condition known as Iliotibial Band (ITB) Syndrome. ITB Syndrome is characterized by pain starting around the hip area, radiating down the outside of the thigh into the outer knee. It is one of the more common causes of leg pain which does not require surgery.

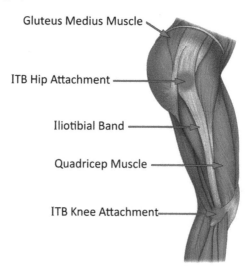

Gluteus Medius Muscle

ITB Hip Attachment

Iliotibial Band

Quadricep Muscle

ITB Knee Attachment

Iliotibial band with hip and knee attachments

The iliotibial band (ITB) is a leg supporting structure. It is a tough, thick band of connective fiber that runs from the outer pelvic bone (hip), down the lateral (outer) part of the thigh and attaches to the tibia bone (shin bone).

At the level of the pelvis, buttocks and hip muscles attach to the ITB. The ITB is a stabilizing band that coordinates the hip and knee function. ITB syndrome is caused by inflammation resulting from this band sliding back and forth across the outer hip bone. This inflammation can spread down the ITB to the knee. If you have ITB syndrome, you may experience pain along the outer thigh down to the knee. This can also cause isolated hip, thigh or knee pain.

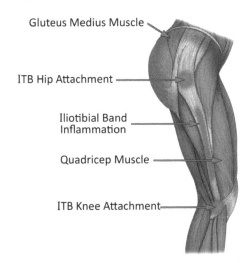

Gluteus Medius Muscle

ITB Hip Attachment

Iliotibial Band Inflammation

Quadricep Muscle

ITB Knee Attachment

ITB inflammation and pain—hip, thigh, knee

ITB syndrome is commonly seen in runners but anyone can develop this condition. Poor flexibility of the quadriceps muscle, hip girdle muscle tightness, leg length inequality, and lack of regular stretching exercises are common causes.

As ITB syndrome progresses, it can mimic a torn meniscus in the knee or even classic sciatic nerve pain. This condition is important to recognize as it is a mechanical problem which requires an entirely different treatment program than knee joint pain or pain coming from the sciatic nerve. ITB syndrome is distinctly not a surgical problem.

It is easily diagnosed by a detailed history and careful physical exam. MRI imaging is not necessary as the physical findings of ITB syndrome are classic, but unfortunately, all too frequently missed or not even considered.

Patients have undergone and failed back (spinal) surgery for sciatica which was actually ITB syndrome, a problem that has nothing to do with the spine.

Because ITB syndrome is a mechanical and inflammatory problem, it should be treated conservatively with anti-inflammatory medications, hands-on physical therapy, and stretching. Acupuncture with a Chinese technique called *gua sha*, can be very effective in treating ITB syndrome. Stretching and strengthening exercises, especially for core muscles, should be done on a daily basis. Prevention is key. Also, good supporting footwear is a must, as is correction of any leg length inequality – another common cause of back pain. Orthotics can be helpful. In more severe cases, Platelet Rich Plasma (PRP) can be used to heal and regenerate the damaged iliotibial band. Surgery should never need to be performed for this condition and runs the risk of making the problem worse or irreversible.

CASE STUDY

Have you heard of "spine fusion?"

"Beth," a 65-year-old patient, was suffering from right hip and upper leg pain. She had seen an orthopedic spine surgeon. She had a lumbar spine MRI scan and was told she had a "bad L5 disc problem." Spine surgery with fusion was scheduled. Fortunately for Beth, she had come to my office for a different problem, but mentioned that she was having back surgery later that week. Careful examination revealed that she actually had severe ITB syndrome and virtually no evidence of any L5 disc problems.

Beth did not go through with the spine fusion, thank goodness. She was treated conservatively, through our office, not for a spine problem, but actually for her ITB syndrome. **She had complete healing and resolution of her pain after three weeks of conservative treatment.**

If you have leg pain that seems like sciatica to you, but runs only from your hip to your knee, you must consider ITB syndrome. The treatment and cure can be conservative and simple. If a doctor recommends surgery for upper leg pain, particularly back surgery, get another opinion.

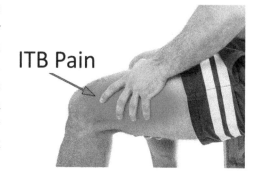

ITB Pain

Piriformis Syndrome

The piriformis muscle plays an important role in symptoms of sciatica. The piriformis muscle attaches at the side of the sacrum and extends horizontally to attach to the upper part of the femur. Although a relatively small muscle, it is one of the main external leg rotator muscles.

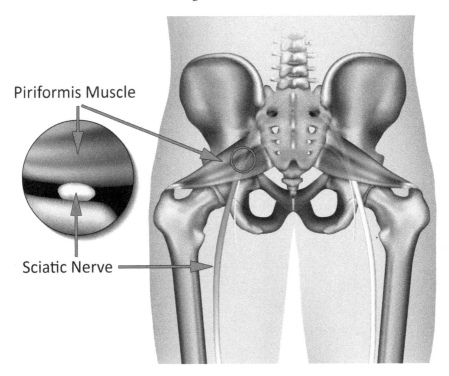

Piriformis Muscle

Sciatic Nerve

Piriformis muscle strain irritates sciatic nerve running under it

A sprain of the piriformis muscle is painful. It causes moderate to severe buttocks pain, made worse by sitting on anything in your back pocket. Anatomically, the sciatic nerve comes out just below or runs through the lower fibers of the piriformis muscle. If the piriformis muscle is injured, strained or inflamed, it can cause irritation to the sciatic nerve. You can have sciatic pain (pain down the leg) with some lower back pain and have nothing wrong with your lumbar spine. The pain is purely coming from the inflamed piriformis muscle with secondary irritation of the sciatic nerve. Piriformis injury healing typically takes weeks to months.

Conservative treatment is the only treatment for Piriformis Syndrome. This would include using ice and daily piriformis and hamstring stretching.

Surgery would never be a consideration—and yet, there are those unfortunate individuals who become victimized by a surgeon who is all too happy to operate to "fix" their sciatica. The entire pelvis with its ligaments, tendons and muscles is a very complex anatomical structure. Injury to many of its muscles, tendons, ligaments and fascia can all result in non-spinal back pain.

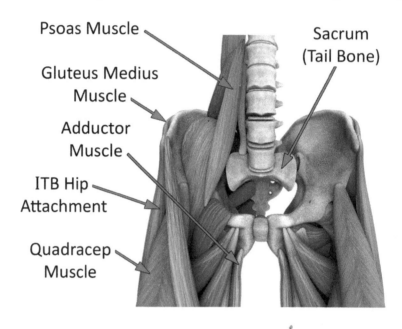

Anterior view of pelvis with muscles attached

CHAPTER 3

Low Back Pain–Pain Without a (Specific) Cause

Why so many ineffective back surgeries? Surgical failure (about 60%) is so prevalent that there is a medical term for it: Failed Back Syndrome (FBS) or Failed Back Surgery Syndrome (FBSS). According to Andrew Milby, M.D., the general definition of Failed Back Surgery Syndrome is "persistent or recurrent symptoms in anybody who has had previous spinal surgery... they might feel like their symptoms never got better, or perhaps even got worse than before. Their symptoms might have gone from back pain to leg pain or from leg pain to back pain, or both."[25]

Over half of all back surgeries are performed for the wrong reason. The mere fact that you have chronic lower back pain is not sufficient to justify any spine surgery.[26] This would explain why there is such a high failure rate of back surgeries in the United States. Published studies have shown that the cause of chronic low back pain is not well defined. In most individuals who suffer from chronic low back pain, it is not possible to identify a specific cause of their pain.[27] Therefore, spine surgery is not at all indicated—how can one operate on a problem, the cause of which cannot even be clearly identified?

If you have low back or neck pain—even if the pain has not responded to conservative therapies—this is not a sufficient reason for spinal surgery. As reported in the *Journal for Neurosurgical Science*, "low back pain (LBP) is a common disorder with a lifetime prevalence of 85%... Only in about 10% of the patients specific underlying disease processes can be identified.." In other words, during your lifetime, you most likely will suffer from one or more episodes of neck or back pain.[28]

The Fitness Factor

A major health problem in the United States and worldwide is obesity. **Being overweight or obese directly contributes to chronic lower back pain.** Our bodies were not designed to carry around an extra 30-100 pounds, or more. Look at it this way—a bag of dog food can weigh 30-50 pounds, a bag of cement, 94 pounds. If you carried around a bag of dog food or cement, all day, every day, you would have complaints about back pain, if you were able to stand or walk. This is what is happening in this country with obesity.

An analogy would be that a pick-up truck would eventually get four blown tires if it was loaded as if it was a dump truck.

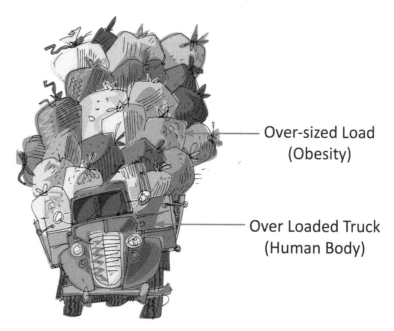

Over-sized Load
(Obesity)

Over Loaded Truck
(Human Body)

*Carrying too much weight (obesity) causes
excessive strain on every part of your body.*

A common cause of chronic lower back pain is poor physical conditioning. With routine daily activities of minimal bending, lifting, stooping, and prolonged sitting, the body becomes deconditioned. Muscles slowly tighten up and start to ache. A flare-up of back pain can occur at any moment with sudden heavy lifting or strain on the back. Something as simple as bending over to tie your shoe, or even a cough or sneeze can be the trigger for acute, painful back muscle spasms.

This is because there was already a problem in your back, and what happened, a sudden strain on your spinal muscles, triggered the flare-up of an already existing back condition. You can have a gradual tightening and weakening of back muscles that do not hurt, but with the wrong movement—bam! Now you have acute, severe lower back pain. Remember, this all has to do with back and hip muscles, tendons, and ligaments. Generally, it has nothing to do with the spine, disc bulges, disc herniations or "pinched" nerve roots.

Rapid weight gain can be even more problematic than the gradual development of obesity. At risk for the onset of back pain caused by lack of muscle strength are women who are pregnant. They can gain a great deal of weight in a relatively short period of time, and it's situated on the front side of their lower back. If they do not have sufficiently strong core muscles, both in the back and abdomen areas, the weight strains the back to a degree that sometimes is incapacitating. The very best way to prevent this, of course, is preconditioning. Using a fitness and exercise routine, a woman can spend at least several months prior to pregnancy to build a stronger frame to handle the weight she will gain. During pregnancy, if she experiences back pain, then stretching, walking, and yoga can be helpful.

Conservative Treatments Can Be Learned and Used by Patients

Acute lower back or neck pain are usually a benign, self-limited problems. Yes, there is pain, but it is not from any ominous cause or spine problem. The vast majority of neck and back pain cases are due to strain on muscles, ligaments, and tendons. They are only rarely related to spinal problems (less than 5%). There is a distinct absence of nerve root symptoms or signs, which may include arm or leg pain with numbness and pain. A detailed history with a careful neurological exam will usually provide the answer as to any serious, underlying problem. Patient education, reassurance, and conservative care should be the first line of care in almost all cases.[29]

It's Never Too Late to Learn

Did you ever have a class in school about how to prevent muscle strain, back pain, or neck problems? Even though we will all experience one or all of these issues at some point in life, we are not taught to understand the meaning, causes, and preventative measures that would be of great help.

These problems can have far-reaching negative effects on mobility, daily activity, and workplace performance. Depending on the severity and duration, these conditions can hinder job performance or prevent us from even going to work, or can force us to change jobs. I see patients who have lost their jobs, lost income, given up golf and other social activities, and even lost relationships due to their aches and pains dictating what they could and could not do. You need to know the risks of remaining uninformed and learn how to keep this from happening to you.

Education, either before you need to see a doctor or once you are a patient, should include instruction on self-care and preventing recurrent episodes of neck or back pain. The latter may include home exercises and/ or hands-on physical therapy. Therapy is to help get tight muscles and fascia stretched out properly. This should be followed by a course of muscle strengthening to "re-balance" all the muscle groups so they are working together. As the founder of Osteopathic Medicine, Dr. A.T. Still, said in 1899, "The fascia is the place to look for the causes of diseases [pain] and the place to begin treatment."

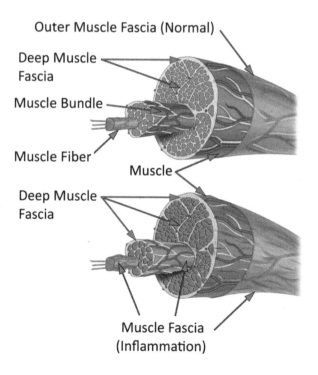

Fascia inflammation, a common cause of "muscle pain"

In the US, low back pain occurs in about 20% of the population, annually.[30] Lifetime prevalence of back pain is 85%.[31] Annual costs for treatment of back and neck pain is in the billions, without even factoring in lost productivity and time missed from work. We can do a better job at changing this dynamic with additional education for the general population as well as for all treating physicians.

MRI scanning is one of the most overutilized diagnostic tests in America. Less than half of the MRI scans ordered for lower back pain have been shown to be appropriate. Unfortunately, the use of MRI scanning is increasing every year. The increasing use of diagnostic imaging does not lead to increases in better health care.[31] If anything, studies have shown that in areas of the country where there is increased use of MRI scanning, the spine surgery rate is higher.[32,33] More back and neck surgery does not equate to better health care, either.

"Only in about 10% of the [back pain] patients can the specific underlying disease processes be identified." Surgery, in these cases, should not be considered the "last option" as it was never an option at all. If there is not a clearly identifiable cause for your back pain (which is very common, over 90%), there should be absolutely no consideration of surgical intervention. Spine surgery should never be "the treatment of last resort if everything else fails."

The concept of exploratory spinal surgery "to see if there is a problem that we can fix" is insanely flawed from the start. Modern day MRI scanning has extraordinarily high resolution for spine and disc abnormalities. If there was a surgically treatable problem causing your pain, it would *clearly* be seen on the MRI images. Do not be persuaded by a spine surgeon into having exploratory spine surgery, especially when your MRI shows no specific problem that would explain your pain. Get a second opinion from a neurologist or physical medicine specialist—somebody who is not a spine surgeon.

Muscles

Muscles of the Back

The Human Spine 1

The spine itself can only support about 35 pounds. It is the many layers of powerful, strong muscles, ligaments and tendons that attach to the spine that allow it to carry around our body mass. No adult weighs only 35 pounds, so the spine requires a lot of assistance if we want to do anything—sit, stand, walk, paddle a kayak, anything. In order for those supporting muscles and tendons to function properly, they must be regularly stretched and strengthened. Maintaining proper balanced muscle strength is critical in the long run to avoid neck and back pain.

Tight muscles naturally become weak. Other muscles then overcompensate for the weaker muscles. This sets up a vicious cycle: the weaker muscles get weaker and the stronger muscles become tighter and more painful. This muscle weakness-tightness cycle is a common cause of neck, upper and lower back pain. That is why regular stretching and strengthening, including core conditioning, is so important for good back health.

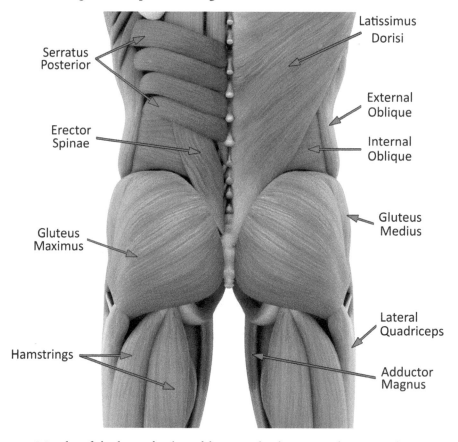

Muscles of the lower back and hips–multiple potential sources of pain

Diagnosis of the majority of cases of lower back or neck pain can be made with a detailed history and careful neurological and musculoskeletal (physical) exam. MRI or CT scans are usually not needed. As previously stated, the findings on scan images rarely demonstrate or explain the cause for the majority of lower back or neck pain cases. **Tight, weak, painful muscles with inflamed fascia cannot be seen on any type of scan.**

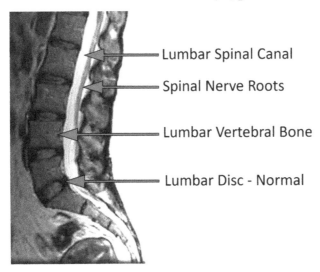

Normal MRI of lumbar spine

Abnormalities Seen on MRI Images Rarely Cause Back Pain

It is common in any given individual, without any back or neck pain symptoms, to have one or more abnormalities on their MRI spine scan. Several studies have shown that up to 70% of individuals without any symptoms will have any combination of disc bulging, disc herniation, arthritic spurs and varying degrees of spinal stenosis—and yet they have no symptoms including pain, numbness or weakness.[34,35] This includes you. If you have no neck or back pain, no symptoms that have you concerned about your spine, there is still a 7 out of 10 chance that your MRI scan will show "abnormalities."[36]

The further along you read in this book, the more convinced you should be that most people do not need spinal surgery. Even when MRI's show significant abnormalities, surgery is not the solution. Why? Because they have no symptoms. You cannot "fix" normal. What the patient and doctor are seeing are merely radiological changes on an MRI study, a picture—that is it. All too many surgeons, doctors, and uninformed patients make the mistake of taking any MRI spinal abnormality (only an imaging finding) and concluding that this is the cause of their pain, or that this means even if there is no pain today, it's just a matter of time. This is *The Great Con.*

The Great Con

Patients are told that they need surgery to correct or "fix" a particular MRI finding as it is the "thing that is causing their pain." Unfortunately, this is a grievously misleading statement. This is using modern technology's amazing scanning capabilities in a dishonest way.

We all know that if an ultrasound image shows a fetus inside a woman's womb, she is definitely pregnant. And an x-ray proves that a bone is broken, or not. So it is not hard to convince people that something visible on an MRI image is "real" and "meaningful." Unfortunately, the fact is that MRI findings are often used by spine institutes as a *marketing technique* to sell the public on the rationalization for back or neck surgery. "If your MRI scan shows an abnormality, we can fix it and relieve your pain." This is *The Big Lie*.

MRI scans, more commonly than not, do not show the cause of neck or back pain—even if there are abnormalities, including disc bulging, disc herniations and varying levels of arthritic (degenerative) changes. Remember, MRI scanning is not necessary or indicated to successfully treat and manage the majority of cases of neck or back pain.

As reported in the *Acta Orthopedic Supplement*: "Chronic low back pain (CLBP) is one of the main causes of disability in the western world with a huge economic burden to society. As yet, no specific underlying anatomic cause has been identified for CLBP. Imaging often reveals degenerative findings of the disc or facet joints of one or more lumbar segments. These findings, however, can also be observed in asymptomatic people...spinal fusion should not be proposed as a standard treatment for chronic low back pain. Causality of nonspecific spinal pain is complex and CLBP should not be regarded as a diagnosis, but rather as a symptom in patients with different stages of impairment and disability."[37]

The World Health Organization lists chronic lower back pain as the #1 worldwide cause of life-years lost to disability.[38]

To Cut or Not to Cut: Rules of Engagement

For clarification on MRI abnormalities, a few rules need to be **strictly** observed when it comes to determining the **need** for spine surgery.

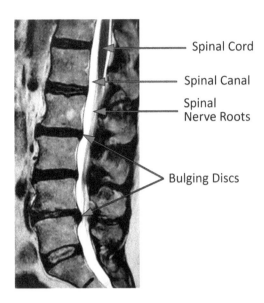

Spinal Cord

Spinal Canal

Spinal
Nerve Roots

Bulging Discs

Bulging discs, lumbar spine—Never require surgery

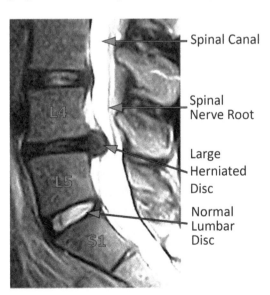

Spinal Canal

Spinal
Nerve Root

Large
Herniated
Disc

Normal
Lumbar
Disc

Large L4-5 lumbar disc herniation

The vertebral discs are the shock absorbers for the spine. A disc consists of 2 main parts: 1) the nucleus, 2) the annulus. The vertebral disc nucleus is a soft, gel-like inner area of the disc. This allows the disc to absorb compression. The annulus is the tough, fibrous outer ring around the nucleus. It maintains the structural integrity of the disc. With repeated trauma and stress over the years, the fibers of the annulus can become weakened. With this, the vertebral disc may have various degenerative changes.

> ## Bulging discs do not cause neck, back, or extremity pain and should NEVER be the reason for spine surgery.

First, annular bulging or disc bulges do not cause symptoms—not neck, back, arm or leg pain. Disc bulging is a common finding in most patients as it is a normal part of your aging spine, developing in your late twenties and continuing through life. This is where the nucleus material is only pushing against the annulus in an area of weakened fibers. Disc bulges should never be operated on.

The next level of disc abnormality is disc protrusions. Disc protrusions are early disc herniations. Depending on severity, they may need surgery. More severe disc protrusions are the similar to a disc herniation, particularly in combination with a congenitally narrow spinal canal. Occasionally, disc protrusions may be close to and compressing an existing nerve root. This may be a reason for surgery, but only if the patient has symptoms corresponding to that particular severe disc protrusion level and clearly has a compressed nerve root, at the same level, with abnormal neurological findings.

Five Types of Disc Degeneration

1. **Degeneration**: The inner gelatinous center pushes into the outer annulus fibrosis, which can cause disc bulging. Seen at all ages. Normal spine aging. Vertebral disc is becoming thinner and dehydrated.

2. **Bulging Disc**: The outer layer of fibrous cartilage around a disc undergoes some degree of degeneration thereby causing a bulging out of the vertebral disc wall. This would be similar to gently squeezing the center of a jelly donut. Bulging discs do not cause symptoms.

3. **Herniation**: The annulus fibrosis forms a protruding bulge or outpouching that sometimes can press against nerves, depending on severity. . Similar to disc protrusion.

   - Lateral Disc Herniation: may compress nerve root
   - Central Disc Herniation: rarely causes symptoms unless severe or extruded

4. **Extrusion**: The annulus fibrosis ruptures but the inner gelatinous center remains intact. This can cause some nerve root compression, due to disc herniation.

5. **Sequestration**: The annulus fibrosis ruptures and the inner gelatinous center separates from the main part of the disc. This is a disc fragment, and is frequently symptomatic.

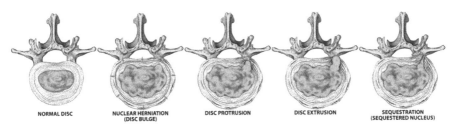

NORMAL DISC   NUCLEAR HERNIATION (DISC BULGE)   DISC PROTRUSION   DISC EXTRUSION   SEQUESTRATION (SEQUESTERED NUCLEUS)

Stages of vertebral disc degeneration

Our Bodies Change Over Time—Aging is Completely Natural

Disc degeneration and bulging is a normal part of the aging spine and should not concern the vast majority of people. This expected type of spinal degeneration essentially does not cause any pain or other symptoms.

While herniated (or extruded) discs *may* be a justification for back surgery, several conditions must first be met. The *critical requirement* is that the location at which the disc is herniated must correlate exactly

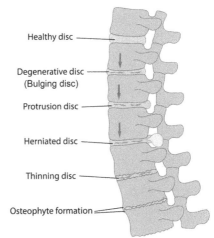

Healthy disc

Degenerative disc (Bulging disc)

Protrusion disc

Herniated disc

Thinning disc

Osteophyte formation

Stages of age-related spine degeneration

with the patient's symptoms of arm or leg pain, numbness and weakness. A herniated disc is almost never the exclusive cause of isolated neck or back pain.

Example: If you have back pain going down the side of your **right** leg, this would suggest anatomically an L_5 lumbar disc problem on your **right** side. If you have a disc herniation at any other level or even at L_5, but to the **left**, this would not cause your symptoms. Why? Because it is at the wrong level, wrong side, or both. Therefore, in this case even with MRI abnormalities, the findings do not explain your symptoms. Even if you do have a disc herniation/extrusion at L_5 on the right, back surgery is not necessarily needed as conservative therapy should be initiated as first line treatment.

Remember, the natural history of symptomatic disc herniation is to heal with conservative therapy in a few weeks.[39] Another important fact is that many individuals have varying degrees of MRI spine abnormalities that cause absolutely no symptoms.[40]

Epidural Steroid Injections: Masking Pain and Making Profit

Epidural steroids are all too commonly prescribed for the treatment of neck and lower back pain. Several published studies[41] have confirmed that epidural steroid treatments are not indicated and are ineffective for most cases of neck and lower back pain, being no more effective than placebo. Why? Epidural injections are intended to be given for treating spine and spinal nerve pain but are also used for generic neck and low back pain. These injections do not heal anything, and at best mask the pain temporarily. Generic back or neck pain do not have a spinal origin but rather most commonly has its origins in the soft tissues components of the neck and back: muscles, tendons, ligaments and fascia (membrane surrounding muscles). ESI treatment universally fails when given for soft tissue back or neck pain.

Inflammation of the soft tissue surrounding the spine: muscles, tendons, ligaments and fascia is the major cause of neck and back pain. This is particularly true for cases of chronic low back pain. Study after study has shown that the specific cause of *chronic* low back pain is vague and not identifiable.

During an epidural steroid injection procedure, a needle is inserted into the spine, usually at the level of the MRI abnormality. The same MRI spinal abnormality that usually has nothing to do with the actual cause of your back or neck pain. The needle is inserted into the area just outside of the spinal sac, known as the epidural space.

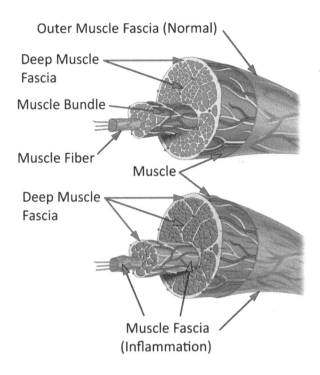

Outer Muscle Fascia (Normal)

Deep Muscle Fascia

Muscle Bundle

Muscle Fiber

Muscle

Deep Muscle Fascia

Muscle Fascia (Inflammation)

Muscle and fascia inflammation causes pain

This is where the term epidural: "epi" *above,* "dural" *fibrous spinal membrane.* Then a mixture of a local anesthetic and steroid is injected into this space. Hence the term "epidural steroid injection." Even in cases of herniated discs, which cause true sciatica, the natural history is to heal on their own. Epidural steroids have been shown in several well-controlled studies to be no more effective than placebo.[42]

In an excellent study published in the *New England Journal of Medicine,* the conclusion was "although epidural injections of methylprednisolone ["steroids"] may afford short-term improvement in leg pain and sensory deficits in patients with sciatica due to a herniated nucleus pulposus ["disc"], this treatment offers no significant functional benefit, nor does it reduce the need for surgery."[43] That is, **if** surgery were even indicated in the first place.

The European medical community has published a great deal of information on the treatment of low back pain. The journal *Schmerz* (German for "pain") released the summarized results of fifteen studies on the effectiveness of epidural steroid injections:

"…these trials showed inconsistent results of epidural injections. Of the 15 trials, 8 reported positive results and 7 others reported negative results. Consequently the efficacy of epidural steroid injections has not yet been established. The benefits of epidural steroid injections seem to be of short duration only… it is unclear which patients benefit from these injections."[44]

The conclusion of another study published in the journal, *Spine*: "There is in sufficient evidence to support the use of injection therapy in sub-acute and chronic low-back pain."[45]

Moreover, epidural steroid injections are not without risk. As noted on the Johns Hopkins medical website, risks include that pain could actually increase. Though rare, other risks are nerve damage, bleeding, allergic reaction, infection, and paralysis.[46] I know of a case where an 82-year-old man asked for and received an epidural injection, and it did temporarily relieve his back pain, but during the procedure he got a staph infection (MRSA) and became seriously ill, contracted pneumonia, and died.

Spinal Cord Stimulators and Other Gimmicks

The number of gimmicks that are actually FDA-approved is quite astounding. For example, radio frequency ablation (known as "rhizotomy") uses electrical current to burn the pain-carrying nerves that come into the spine. While this procedure is frequently not effective for long-term back or neck pain control, physicians continue to heap this money-making procedure on the unsuspecting public. At best, you can expect short term pain relief—weeks to a couple of months. At worst, it will be a useless procedure that sets you back a few thousand dollars.

Spinal cord stimulators are another pain control scheme. In this procedure, an implantable spine stimulator (pacemaker-like device) is surgically placed under the skin. The electrodes are placed so that the dorsal nerve root tracts (*pain nerves*) in the spine are stimulated. The dorsal nerve columns in your spinal cord control pain impulse transmission. Block these columns and pain will theoretically be stopped. While this may sound good in theory, the failure rate of spinal cord stimulation is not low (about 20%, or 1 out of 5). Failure is common and includes lack of pain control, infection, electrodes breaking or moving, dead battery and device malfunction. This combined with a high complication rate of up to 40%, make it a poor choice for management of pain from Failed Back Syndrome.[47,48]

It Is Unlikely that Your Spine Is the Cause of Your Pain

The *vast majority of neck and back pain is due to soft tissue injury of some type*—muscle, tendon, fascia, ligament. The pain is not originating from the spine or nerve roots coming out of the spine. Doing an epidural injection or radio frequency ablation for non-spinal pain is exposing you to an unnecessary, invasive procedure and the complications that go with this. Complications can include infection, spinal cord and permanent nerve root damage.

> ### The vast majority of neck and back pain is due to soft tissue injury.

This is supported by another study published in the *Annals of Internal Medicine*, entitled: "Nonpharmacologic Therapies for Acute and Chronic Low Back Pain: A review of the evidence for an American Pain Society/ American College of Physicians Clinical Practice Guideline." Here is the conclusion: "Therapies with good evidence of moderate efficacy for chronic or sub-acute low back pain are cognitive-behavioral therapy, exercise, spinal manipulation, and interdisciplinary rehabilitation."[49] No injections, no ablations, no implants, no surgery.

We have discussed the natural history of neck and back pain as well as disc herniation, which is to heal with conservative therapy in a few weeks. All patients with back and/or leg pain should be treated with conservative, non-invasive therapy first and foremost.

Spine Surgery Can Only Accomplish Two Things:

1. Decompress a nerve root or spinal cord that is being severely compressed (OR)
2. Stabilize a painful spine joint segment

That is it. That is the sum total of what spine surgery can possibly do.

Nothing more than that.

If you do not have one of these two specific conditions, you do not need spine surgery, period. Be wary of any spine surgeon who promises a "cure" for your back or neck pain, wants to rush into do surgery before "something serious happens" or those that suggest "exploratory spine surgery" to look for a problem. These are all serious red flags that are telling you to find another doctor. Remember, spine surgery is generally an elective procedure.

Essentially 99% of the time, it is never an emergency. You have time to consider your options, do your research and get a different (preferably non-surgical) opinion.

A German study concludes: "…low back pain is a very common symptom. Up to 90% of all adults suffer at least once in their life from a low back pain episode, in the majority of cases a nonspecific lumbago. They are, with or without sciatica, usually self-limited and have no serious underlying pathology and subside in 80-90% of the [affected] patients within six weeks. Beside a sufficient pain medication and physiotherapy, reassurance about the overall benign character and the favorable prognosis of the medical condition should be in the center of the therapeutic efforts. In a multimodal therapeutic concept, the patient education should focus on the natural history of an acute back pain episode, the overall good prognosis, and recommendations for an effective [non-surgical] treatment."[50] A similar American study, with the same conclusions, was published in the journal, *American Family Physician.*[51] In other words, studies and science confirm that the typical sources of back and neck pain will be resolved by the body, over time, especially with the assistance of non-surgical, conservative therapy.

Other MRI spinal abnormalities that may be seen include spinal stenosis and slippage of one vertebra on the other, a condition known as "spondylolisthesis." There are different degrees of both of these conditions. There is spinal stenosis and then there is *severe* spinal stenosis. Many cases of spinal stenosis, which is arthritic narrowing of the spinal canal, never need to be treated surgically. Unless a patient has severe leg pain when walking distances of a block or less (claudication), spinal surgery for lumbar stenosis is usually not indicated.

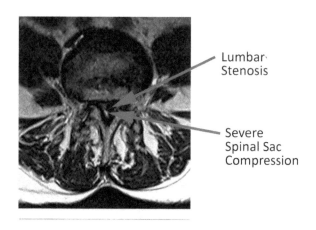

Lumbar Stenosis

Severe Spinal Sac Compression

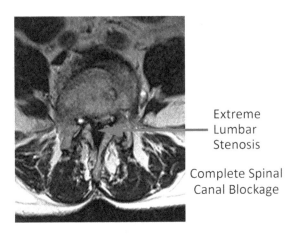

Extreme Lumbar Stenosis

Complete Spinal Canal Blockage

CASE STUDY

"Sharon" is a 66-year-old female who had a lumbar spine MRI for nonspecific, intermittent low back pain. The MRI showed only severe stenosis at the L4-5 level. She did not have any leg pain or claudication. Claudication is pain in the legs with walking, which clears with sitting. I had reviewed her MRI scan, confirming the severe stenosis. Surgery was not recommended as she had virtually no symptoms. Extremely severe stenosis, yet no symptoms. A few years later, Sharon came back into my office. She now had complaints of leg pain with walking, which would clear with rest—claudication. She now had symptomatic spinal stenosis. Sharon had a routine spinal decompression surgery, to relieve the pressure on the spinal cord. She recovered well and has been pain-free ever since. Spine surgery done for the right reason with the right procedure can yield a favorable outcome.

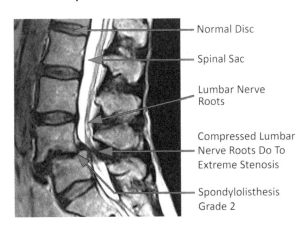

Normal Disc

Spinal Sac

Lumbar Nerve Roots

Compressed Lumbar Nerve Roots Do To Extreme Stenosis

Spondylolisthesis Grade 2

Severe lumbar spinal stenosis with Grade 2 spondylolisthesis

Spondylolisthesis Stages

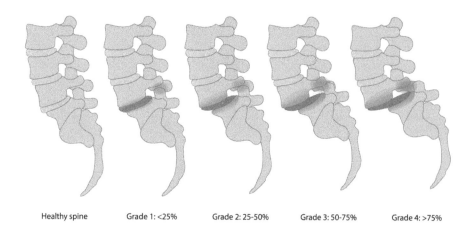

| Healthy spine | Grade 1: <25% | Grade 2: 25-50% | Grade 3: 50-75% | Grade 4: >75% |

Stages of lumbar spondylolisthesis (vertebral slippage).

Careful—You May Need Special Treatment

Let's look at some additional instances where surgery may be justified. In your neck (cervical spine) a lesser degree of stenosis *may* suggest the need for surgery. If there is any degree of spinal cord compression in the neck, surgery should be carefully considered. The reason is that if you were to have any type of whiplash injury, it could temporarily make the existing stenosis momentarily worse. An analogy would be that when bending a garden hose, the inner diameter becomes constricted and smaller.

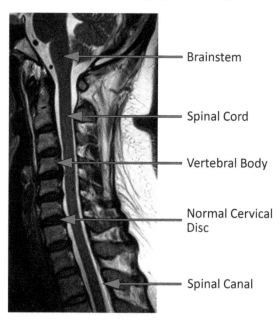

Normal MRI cervical spine

This can result in direct trauma to the spinal cord, resulting in bruising and/or damage to the cord. This may cause weakness in the arms and legs.

The most severe form, quadriplegia, could be the outcome. This type of problem does not exist in the lumbar spine. Stenosis in the cervical spine of less than 9 millimeters (mm) may require surgical treatment.

CASE STUDY

"Vicky" is a 57-year-old woman who had headaches and nonspecific neck pain for many years. Her headaches were well-controlled, but her neck pain would come and go. Her neurological exam was normal. On one visit, Vicky indicated that while her neck pain was not bothering her, she had developed a feeling of weakness in her right hand. Her exam showed some forearm numbness and subtle right grip weakness. Key neurological finding: **numbness and weakness**.

An MRI cervical spine scan was ordered, showing moderately severe cervical spinal stenosis, at the correct level which would cause grip weakness. Neurosurgical consultation was requested. Vicky underwent cervical spinal cord decompression surgery for the spinal stenosis. She made a full and complete recovery.

Generally, to be symptomatic, lumbar (low back) stenosis of the diameter of the spinal canal of less than 4 mm is required. Smaller is worse. Slippage of one vertebra on the other (*spondylolisthesis*) occurs in varying degrees. It is a forward displacement of a vertebra over a lower vertebra, due to a congenital defect or injury. There are four grades of spondylolistheses.

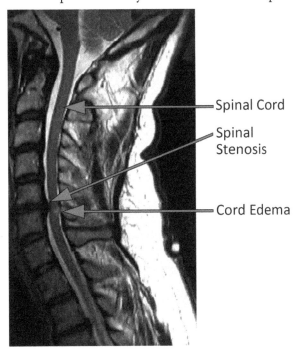

Cervical spinal stenosis with spinal cord compression and edema—surgery required

Grades 1 and 2 generally do not need surgery. In some cases of Grades 3 and 4 spondylolisthesis, surgery may be justified—if the findings explain and directly correlate with the patient's symptoms and neurological findings. Spondylolisthesis can make spinal stenosis worse.

> ## The natural history of disc herniation is to heal with conservative therapy within a few weeks.

Unless combined with severe spinal stenosis or other spinal abnormalities causing severe traction on and/or compression of the spinal nerve roots or spinal cord, surgery is not indicated.

Cauda Equina Syndrome

A relatively rare condition known as "cauda equina syndrome" is caused by severe compression of the lowest end of the spinal cord. The trailing nerve roots at the end of the spinal cord are known as the *cauda equina* or "horses tail." Severe compression of the cauda equina can be caused by severe spinal stenosis, massive disc herniation, tumor, or trauma with fracture at the level of the cauda equina. Symptoms include severe lower back pain, pain in one or both legs, numbness of the pelvic region ("saddle anesthesia"), loss of bowel/bladder control, and leg weakness with gait abnormalities. True cauda equina syndrome is considered a neurological emergency that requires urgent medical evaluation and treatment. Emergency spinal cord decompression surgery is the only treatment for this condition, to avoid permanent neurological deficit.

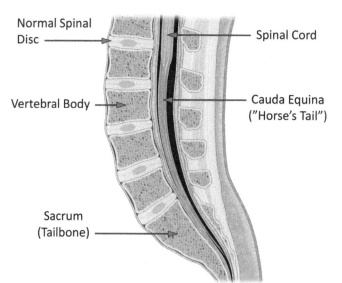

Normal Spinal Disc — Spinal Cord

Vertebral Body — Cauda Equina ("Horse's Tail")

Sacrum (Tailbone)

The collection of nerves at the end of the spinal cord is known as the cauda equina, due to its resemblance to a horse's tail.

The spinal cord ends at the upper portion of the lumbar (lower back) spine.

CASE STUDY

"Heather," a 40-year-old female, suffered from lower back pain. The pain persisted and then suddenly became severe. Within days, she developed numbness of her pelvic region with pain going down the back of both legs. She had some slight difficulty urinating. Her legs felt weak. An emergency MRI was done of her lumbar spine. This showed a large, extruded disc herniation compressing the very end of the cauda equina.

Heather underwent emergency back surgery the very next morning, to decompress the cauda equina. Her recovery was uneventful and the majority of her neurological deficits cleared. She was left with only a slight degree of numbness in the pelvic region.

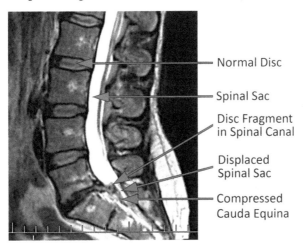

Cauda equina compression 1

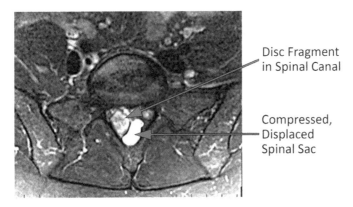

Cauda equina compression 2

Before considering surgery, a patient should have MRI findings of spinal stenosis associated with nerve root compression, spinal cord compromise, and clinical signs and symptoms.

Summary/Conclusion/Action Items

In summary, consider the following facts about MRI findings:

- **Disc bulges:** do not cause pain symptoms—they are the result of any aging spine.

- **Spinal stenosis:** Of mild, moderate, and severe, only severe lumbar stenosis may be symptomatic causing leg claudication which is pain with walking. In the neck, stenosis may cause arm numbness or weakness and your ability to walk normally could be compromised.

- **Disc herniation**

    - Central – usually asymptomatic

    - Lateral – May cause symptoms if severe

    - Herniation with Fragment – usually symptomatic

    - Arthritic Spurs (Osteophytes) – usually no symptoms

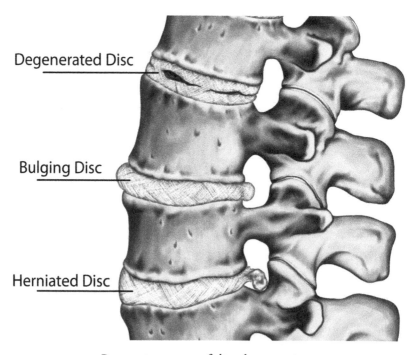

Degenerated Disc

Bulging Disc

Herniated Disc

Progressive stages of disc degeneration

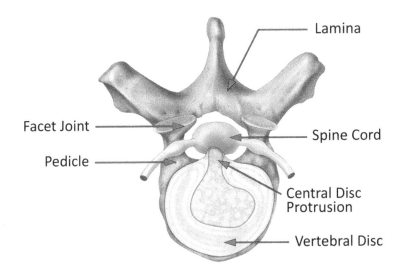

Central disc herniation—usually not symptomatic

MRI findings alone are NOT sufficient to justify spine surgery

Again, spine surgery only accomplishes two possible things:

- Decompress a nerve root or spinal cord that is being severely compressed.
- Stabilize a painful spine joint segment.

Unless one of these two specific problems is causing your pain, you do not need spine surgery.

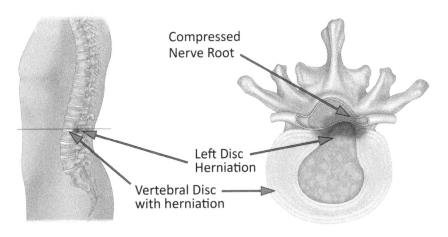

Left-sided herniated disc, compressing nerve root

Spinal Canal
Normal

Spinal Cord

Cervical Nerve
Root

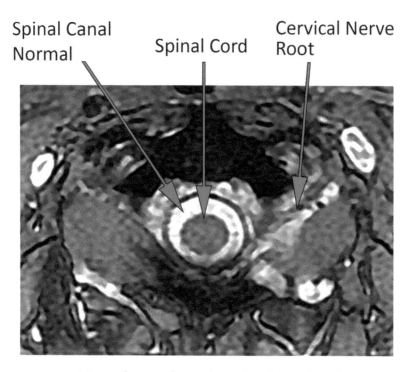

Normal cervical spinal canal and spinal cord

Vertebral Body
Arthritic Spur

Spinal Cord
Compression

Cervical Nerve
Root

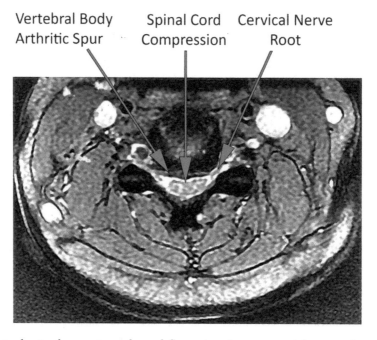

Cervical spinal stenosis with cord flattening (compare with normal image)

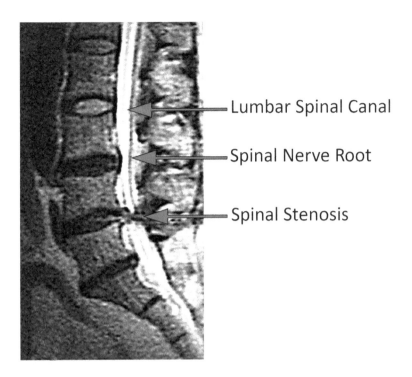

Lumbar Spinal Canal

Spinal Nerve Root

Spinal Stenosis

Lumbar spinal stenosis—severe

CASE STUDY

"Steve" is a now 55-year-old man who suffers from disabling back pain. He had had a history of recurrent episodes of low back pain with left leg sciatica for a few years prior. One day, he was putting a box of items in the backseat of his car. When he bent over to do this, he felt "a strange pop" in his lower back—like he had never felt before. Associated with this was acute low back pain with an electrical pain sensation running down the back of his left leg.

The pain persisted and progressively worsened. He developed a slight left foot drop and change in his gait. Steve would have an occasional fall, from catching his left foot. He had never fallen before. After only a few weeks of pain and leg weakness, he sought out medical help. A detailed exam was performed, showing a left foot drop and some sensory loss that suggested an L5 nerve root compression. This was confirmed after an MRI lumbar spine was performed. The scan showed a large disc herniation with a free disc fragment in the spinal canal. The disc fragment was severely compressing his left L5 nerve root. Back surgery was performed days later. While he had some relief, his foot drop persisted as did his back pain. The leg pain was better.

Steve was eager to return to work after only two weeks following surgery, not allowing sufficient time for healing. Shortly thereafter, his back and leg pain worsened. He tried medications and physical therapy without relief. A second MRI lumbar spine was performed three months after his surgery. This showed another large disc herniation at the same level as before. Steve did not want another surgery so he continued with conservative treatment, being careful not to overexert himself. Despite this the pain persisted and slowly worsened.

He had his second back surgery two years after the first. This time, he not only had the disc fragment removed but also a fusion. Following this surgery, he rested and did back rehabilitation for three months. After this, Steve returned to work. He continued working for about eight months, but his back pain slowly worsened as did his leg pain. He had trouble walking due to foot drop and numbness. Multiple falls were a problem. He had to stop working again.

A third back MRI scan was performed. This showed a disc herniation at the L4 level with a significant Grade 2 spondylolisthesis at L5-S1, causing severe nerve root compression. He tried more conservative therapy in order to avoid another back surgery. Eventually, he became unable to do even the lightest physical activity without setting off disabling back pain. He started using

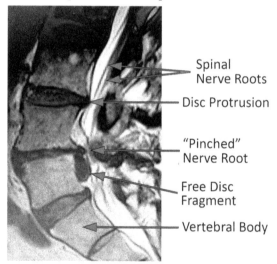

Spinal Nerve Roots

Disc Protrusion

"Pinched" Nerve Root

Free Disc Fragment

Vertebral Body

Lumbar disc herniation free fragment

a motorized scooter, as prolonged standing or walking only made his pain worse. Three years after his second back surgery, he could not take the intractable pain any longer. He had his third back surgery. This included a partial disc removal, fusion and pedicle screws with rods.

Finally he had pain relief. His leg pain cleared but the foot drop and numbness did not. He continues to have variable degrees of back pain, exacerbated with even light physical activity. Unfortunately, he remains permanently disabled to this day. The following are images of his first MRI back scan:

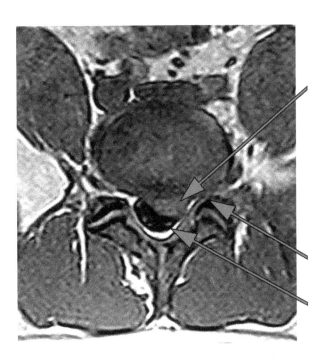

Disc Fragment in Spinal Canal

Compressed Nerve Root

Displaced Spinal Sac

Large, extruded lumbar disc herniation free fragment—needs surgery

Steve's story shows that not all back surgery, even when done for all the right reasons by highly skilled neurosurgeons, has a good outcome. Back surgery, even when indicated, is clearly not without significant risk.

"A healthy body is a guest chamber for the soul; a sick body is a prison."

—Francis Bacon

CHAPTER 4

MRI Abnormalities: Fake Reason for Pain

Back pain is generally not caused by spine or disc problems which are commonly seen on MRI and CT scans. As noted in the introduction, your lower back pain—and neck pain, for that matter—is not caused by spinal or disc problems. Muscles and other soft tissue support structures in these areas (such as tendons, ligaments and fascia) are subject to great stresses and strains as a normal part of daily living, and must not be overlooked as the main source of pain. Fascia is the outer wrapping of connective tissue around muscles. Fascia actually wraps around all muscles, internal organs and virtually everything inside your body. It provides tissue strength and allows a low friction surface for everything to move around. Muscle fascia contains many pain fibers. Fascia strain is a very common cause of "back muscle pain."

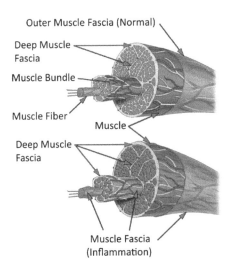

Outer Muscle Fascia (Normal)
Deep Muscle Fascia
Muscle Bundle
Muscle Fiber
Muscle
Deep Muscle Fascia
Muscle Fascia (Inflammation)

Muscle and fascia strain with inflammation

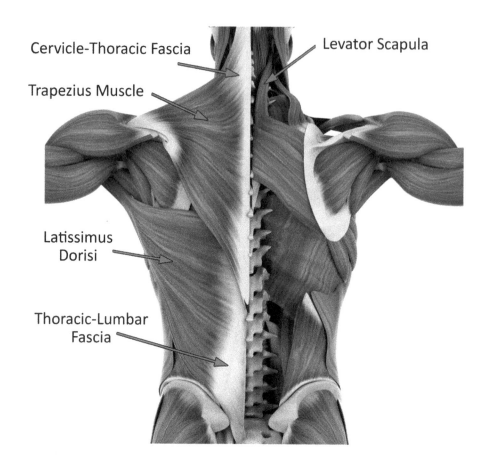

Cervicle-Thoracic Fascia

Levator Scapula

Trapezius Muscle

Latissimus Dorisi

Thoracic-Lumbar Fascia

Spinal muscle outer fascia

We have all "slept wrong" and woke up with a pain in our neck. This usually clears within a few hours or days at the most. Overexertion, doing heavy lifting, yard work, or even exercising too much can strain the back muscles and cause lower back pain. This is compounded by the fact that most Americans have poor back conditioning, poor core conditioning, and are "out of shape."

Unfortunately, obesity and sedentary lifestyles have become endemic in the United States. This is a recipe for disaster when it comes to not only neck or back pain, but other conditions such as diabetes, high blood pressure, high cholesterol, and heart disease. Sitting is clearly the new smoking—it has become a common, daily habit that people don't think much about, unaware of how detrimental it is to their health.

Sitting is the new smoking…it is dangerous!

Advertisements abound for products and diets to rid us of "stubborn belly fat," but this issue is much more serious than only having us avoid wearing a swimsuit in public. Fat around the midsection is a strong risk factor for heart disease, type-2 diabetes, and even some types of cancers.[52,53] And then there is the bad news that belly fat means big trouble for your poor back.

Central obesity (excessive abdominal fat around the stomach and abdomen) causes the pelvis to tilt forward, resulting in added tension on the spine. This pulls on the muscles of the back to maintain body stabilization. These muscles, under a great deal of stress, are prone to sprains and strains—the most common cause of back pain. There is a direct correlation between obesity and accelerated knee joint degeneration and arthritic changes.[54]

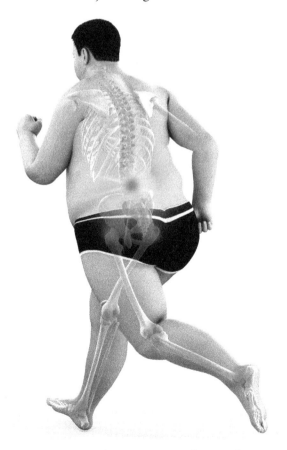

Lower back, hip, knee pain due to obesity

Maybe it's Arthritis?

It is uncommon for arthritic changes in the mid to lower spine to cause pain symptoms. In contrast, cervical (neck) arthritis, if moderate or severe, can cause neck pain of varying degrees. This, however, is not a reason to undergo neck surgery. Generally, in affected individuals, the arthritic changes are at multiple levels and no one area can be identified as the specific origin of your pain. This condition is known as "cervical degenerative disease." Spine surgery on the neck for general arthritis can make your pain worse. The treatment for this is taking anti-inflammatory agents, ice, moist heat, acupuncture, and occasional therapeutic massage.

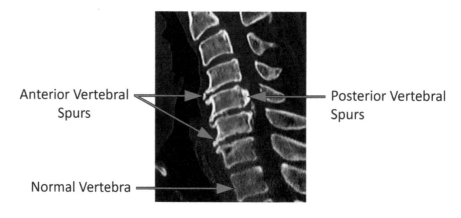

Anterior Vertebral Spurs

Posterior Vertebral Spurs

Normal Vertebra

Cervical arthritic changes and spurs

CHAPTER 5

The MRI Scan is Lying About Your Neck and Back Pain

Over a lifetime, almost all Americans (9 out of 10) will develop various spine and vertebral disc abnormalities, which are seen on MRI scans, *which produce no symptoms.* MRI scan spine abnormalities are common and are not a reason to see a spine surgeon to have neck or back surgery.[55]

> ### An MRI simply cannot tell you that surgery is the solution.

By the age of 30, our spines start undergoing normal degenerative changes—changes due to the wear and tear of daily living. For an aging spine, it is normal to be abnormal. It is frequently as benign as having your hair turn grey.

Of course, this varies from individual to individual for a multitude of reasons including genetics, level of physical conditioning, type of employment, level of physical activity, sports played, and history of recurrent physical trauma. The latter is a major reason that professional football players are plagued by early onset of symptomatic arthritis.

The normal, age-related developments of spinal degenerative changes do not mean that any of these will cause, or is the cause of, neck or back pain. The changes—arthritic spurring, bulging discs, mild spinal stenosis and even disc herniation—are all natural processes of aging. The fact that these changes are apparent on MRI scanning does not in any way mean that they are causing any pain, numbness, weakness or any other symptoms.

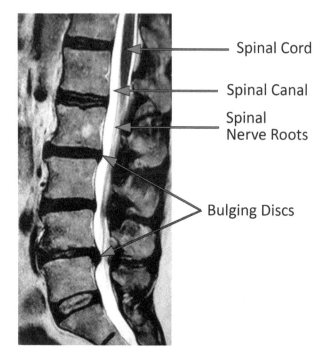

Spinal Cord

Spinal Canal

Spinal
Nerve Roots

Bulging Discs

Spine disc bulging—not a source of pain

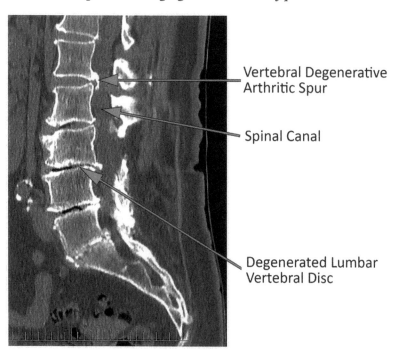

Vertebral Degenerative
Arthritic Spur

Spinal Canal

Degenerated Lumbar
Vertebral Disc

Lumbar spine arthritic (degenerative) changes

Unfortunately, an MRI scan is often used as visual "evidence" by spinal surgeons or pain management specialists, looking for an obvious sign of a physical x-ray change that could be blamed as the source of pain. Many surgeons misinterpret (or misrepresent) MRI changes in the spine as the primary causes of your neck or back pain. As published in the *Current Review of Musculoskeletal Medicine*: "There is limited role of [MRI] imaging in non-specific acute low back pain without the red flags, as the [MRI] findings correlate poorly with symptoms."[56] The general public has been led down the primrose path of this all-too-common misconception: any *MRI abnormality equals the cause of your pain*, and this error is used frequently and incorrectly to justify doing spine surgery.[57]

Flawed conclusions of MRI images showing spine abnormalities associated with normal aging is a common reason for unnecessary neck or back surgery. For example, a patient has back pain with or without leg pain, the MRI spine shows one or more "abnormalities," the patient has surgery based solely on the MRI changes —merely a picture of the spine. Unless the MRI findings correlate precisely with the neurological exam abnormalities and explain your symptoms, the changes seen on your MRI study are not the cause of your pain. This is usually the case, whether a surgeon is saying it, or not.[58] "No proof can be found for the benefit of surgery in patients with low back pain, without [having] serious neurologic deficit."

CASE STUDY

Cindy, a 30-year-old realtor, had a history of head and neck pain. Her headaches were treated conservatively and came under control without the use of pain killers. Her neck pain was nonspecific in nature, due to underlying soft tissue pain. Various noninvasive and non-narcotic treatments were tried. Although her neck pain improved, it did not clear. A friend of hers suggested that she come to see me after she received the alarming news from her doctor that she needed neck surgery.

That doctor had ordered an MRI cervical spine study on Cindy, and then she was told that she needed neck surgery. Cindy had neck pain only, without arm pain, weakness, or numbness. Her neurological exam was completely normal. I reviewed her MRI scan in detail with her. The study showed only minimal arthritic degenerative changes and a minor disc bulge. It was clear that **her current pain was not related to the MRI findings**. I told her to not let anyone operate on her neck, as this would not help her, warning her that she could end up permanently worse off. Soon after this, Cindy became pregnant and did not follow up with me about her neck pain due to insurance issues.

She returned to our clinic about two years later, now with severe, debilitating neck pain. She had undergone neck surgery only a few months before and now was having more pain than ever. She wanted us to "do something about my neck pain. "Fix it." I reviewed the second MRI scan she had had. This study was not any different than the first study we had reviewed with her two years earlier. Specifically, the second study was normal for her age, and clearly there was no spine abnormality that would have caused her pain. Here is another victim of unnecessary neck surgery. Now a 34-year old mother with a small child, poor Cindy had Failed Neck Surgery Syndrome. She could no longer work and had to go on disability. Thirty-four-years-old and on disability for life!

Remember, for the right or (more commonly) wrong reasons, spine surgery is not reversible. Do not fall into this trap. Cindy had a minor asymptomatic disc bulge that was operated on with a fusion spine surgery, with a permanent and disastrous outcome.

Rain Dancing

We can look at the other side of the equation. In the case of a symptomatic disc herniation, conservative therapy is still the indicated first line therapy as the natural history of herniated discs is to heal on their own, over a few weeks.

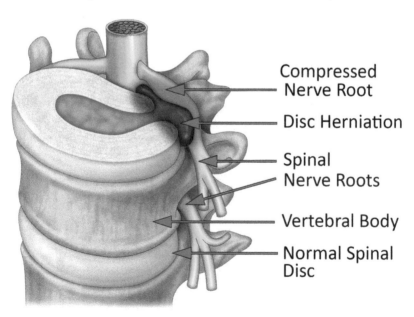

Compressed Nerve Root

Disc Herniation

Spinal Nerve Roots

Vertebral Body

Normal Spinal Disc

Left disc herniation compressing exiting nerve root

Several studies have been done looking at the MRI spine findings of individuals with absolutely no history of neck or back pain. Totaling all the studies, a 2015 review of several thousand of these individuals had MRI study imaging which was summarized.[59]

> ### 70% of individuals with no history of pain will have MRI spine abnormalities.

The findings in these studies were that there are MRI spinal abnormalities in up to 7 out of 10 individuals—people with no history of having any pain at all. *Seventy percent!* That means that there are 230 million U.S. citizens walking around with significant MRI or CT abnormalities with virtually no symptoms of neck, back, arm, or leg pain. MRI imaging abnormalities found included disc bulging, disc protrusion, disc herniation, spinal stenosis, and varying degrees of arthritic changes. Obviously, no experienced, knowledgeable, ethical physician would suggest to these individuals, without them having any symptoms and normal neurological exam, that they undergo spinal surgery. Perhaps if you were handsomely compensated to do a rain dance because the ground was dry, you would dance and hope for rain. But, just like MRI findings and your pain, there is simply no real correlation.

You cannot fix what is not broken

Again, the findings of the normal processes of any aging spine, including yours, are not sufficient justification for surgical intervention. This is one of the most common reasons for inappropriate and unnecessary neck or back surgery and the resultant high failure rate of spine surgery, leading to a condition known as Failed Back Syndrome or Post-Laminectomy Syndrome, i.e., persistent or worse neck or back pain following spine surgery.

> ### Failed Back Syndrome is most commonly the result of inappropriate spine surgery.

The horrible truth is that the pain after surgery can be, and frequently is, worse than before the surgery. Surgery is a one way process. You cannot do a second surgery to "fix" the first surgical failure. Remember Cindy's story. To conclude, just because the MRI scan shows one or more abnormalities, as it commonly does, this does not necessarily explain the cause of your neck or back pain.

The illustration below shows what a typical spine fusion outcome looks like. The procedure involves using metal screws, rods, and a fusion cage. This hardware sometimes causes more problems, especially if the screws are placed improperly or, after a time, they sometimes break. A broken pedicle screw frequently means additional spine surgery.

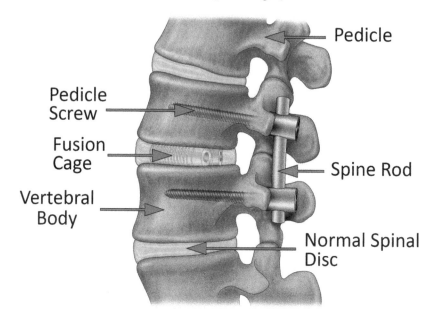

Spinal hardware: pedicle screws with spinal rodding and fusion cage

"I will consider the benefit of my patient and abstain from whatever is deleterious and mischievous."

—from The Hippocratic Oath

CHAPTER 6

Back Surgery Complications—Death is Not Reversible

Millions of people have benefitted from the "miracles of modern medicine," as healthcare is often called today because of the dramatic increase in effective treatments available now versus just a few decades ago. Modern healthcare in the US improves countless lives every single day; however, it is not without risk. We have learned to expect "miracles" and discuss endlessly the ways our loved ones and ourselves have benefitted through medical procedures, new prescription drugs, and innovative treatments. Because of the successes we have come to expect, it is shocking when we hear of failures, and of course, of how many deaths every year result from Western medical care. 225,000 deaths are reported and of these, there are:

- 12,000 from unnecessary surgery
- 7,000 from medication errors in hospitals
- 20,000 from other errors in hospitals
- 80,000 from infections in hospitals
- 106,000 from non-error, negative effects of drugs[60]

Since almost all back surgeries are performed in hospitals or spine centers, you can conclude that **some percentage of the annual hospital and unnecessary surgery deaths cited above are related to spine surgeries.** Do not be one of the 12,000 unnecessary death-from-surgery victims. Death is not reversible. Beware that if you undergo any surgery, you are exposing yourself to all the other potential fatal complications above.

Laser vs. Scalpel: Both are Complicated and Precarious

Besides death, other complications of back surgery are all too common. During back surgery, the surgeon is cutting down to the spine and disc area. Whether it is with a scalpel or laser, the procedure is essentially the same. This means that laser spine surgery offers little, if any, advantage over conventional, minimally invasive spine surgery. The spinal nerves are exiting the spine in the area of the surgical procedure and are exposed to risk of injury either from scalpel or laser.

> **Laser spine surgery has the same risk of nerve damage as comparable conventional surgery.**

Vast marketing campaigns have been used to sell people on laser spine surgery, leading to many people having interest based on wrong ideas. "People think a laser beam shoots through their skin and their pain is gone," S. Kurpad, MD, said in an article published by the Medical College of Wisconsin. "But, as with other minimally invasive techniques…there is an incision involved in laser spine surgery, too. There is also a greater risk of damaging nerves or tissue with a laser, and most importantly, there is no scientific evidence to suggest laser spine surgery is in any way superior to a non-laser approach."[61]

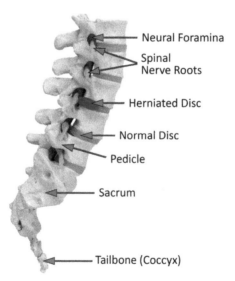

Neural Foramina

Spinal Nerve Roots

Herniated Disc

Normal Disc

Pedicle

Sacrum

Tailbone (Coccyx)

Lumbar spine model showing nerve roots and herniated disc at L3-4

Your spinal nerves can easily be damaged during surgical procedures, particularly when operating on more than one spine level. The risk of nerve damage with a multiple level surgery ranges from 5-20%. Pain is the most common consequence of this. Prior back/neck surgeries, smoking, and obesity dramatically increase these risks further.[62] "Laser discectomy may be more effective in attracting patients than in treating them."[63]

There is a high correlation with smoking and bad outcomes. Smoking leads to poor blood supply to the discs and vertebrae, ultimately ending in poor results for back or neck surgery.[64] Smoking impairs healing after any surgery, but studies have shown that is particularly true in cases of back surgery. Blood supply into the spinal bones is already limited. Smoking further limits fresh, oxygen rich blood from getting into the spine, thereby delaying and interfering with complete healing. In smokers, surgical failures and complications are much higher.[65]

Why You Want to Avoid Nerve Damage

By the way, all you need to perform spine surgery is a medical license—you do not have to be a trained surgeon. This can make the consequences of adverse effects even more serious. According to a 2016 study published in Surgical Neurology International, more and more frequently, the physicians performing laser disc decompression surgeries are not surgeons, but instead, "pain management specialists" like anesthesiologists, radiologists, or physiatrists. The researcher says "the laser vaporizes/shrinks a small portion of disc tissue that lowers intradiscal pressure/volume, and thereby provides symptomatic relief but the surgeries were "ineffective for managing acute/chronic pain in these patients." Without surgical training, the pain management specialists were unable to address surgical complications.[66]

> ## Once a nerve is damaged,
> ## it may never completely heal.

Once your spinal nerve is damaged, it may or may not heal. If it does heal, this may be incomplete. The end result is that you have the same or more pain and may end up with more neurological deficits, either persistent numbness or weakness such as foot drop, or leg or arm weakness. Nerve damage is frequently not reversible, particularly in the case of pain and numbness. There is no effective treatment for any type of numbness or loss of sensation.

Nerve damage not only can present as persistent numbness or weakness, but can have other clinical symptoms as well. One of these is *neurogenic bladder*. In this condition, the nerves to the urinary bladder are damaged. Patients undergoing spinal surgery can develop neurogenic bladder, resulting in not being able to urinate voluntarily. Affected patients will need to catheterize themselves for the rest of their life. This condition is not reversible. Another way the bladder can be affected by nerve damage is the onset of *urinary incontinence*—the inability to stop urine from coming out. Lifetime adult diapers could be the only answer.

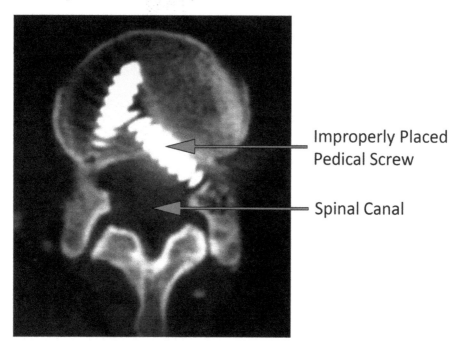

Improperly Placed Pedical Screw

Spinal Canal

Poorly placed pedicle screw—compromising spinal canal.

Another more radical form of nerve damage involves sexual function. As a complication of spinal surgery, **men can lose their ability to get an erection.** This condition is known as *erectile dysfunction*. **Erectile dysfunction due to nerve damage cannot be treated with drugs like Viagra® or Cialis®.** Since the nerves cannot be repaired, more surgery is needed to correct the problem with a mechanical penile implant. Surgical correction of neurogenic erectile dysfunction may include placing an implantable penis balloon, to simulate an erection.

Sexual dysfunction can result for women, as well, due to nerve damage. Women can permanently lose the ability to orgasm, due to damage of the delicate nerves involved in this normal, human function. There is no medical treatment for this.

Infection and Consequences

Infection is another all too common complication of back (and other) surgeries. The rate of infection is generally about one percent. Some surgeons have higher infection rates, perhaps 2-3%. Developing an infection after spinal surgery is a very serious problem. It requires prolonged courses of antibiotics, leaving the body more vulnerable and potentially causing antibiotic resistance. If an abscess develops, more surgery is needed to drain this. With a severe infection, it can take months to clear up and other complications can set in. This can also result in more persistent pain and worsening of the pain syndrome.

Of all US hospital admissions, 5 % of the patients come out with an infection they did not have when they went in.

Centers for Disease Control (CDC) reports there were an estimated 1.7 million healthcare-associated infections and almost 100,000 deaths from those infections in 2002. Even today, hospital acquired infections remain a major problem. If you have spine surgery, you are subjecting yourself to these potentially fatal infection risks.

Persistent Pain

Persistent pain following back or neck surgery is common and may be due to any number of causes. First and foremost, spine surgery was never indicated and had virtually no possibility of eliminating neck or back pain. Secondarily, the surgery itself causes scar tissue to form around the nerve roots. Spinal hardware such as pedicle screws, put in to stabilize the spine, can cause pain. These screws are placed into the vertebral bodies to secure metal plates or other hardware. Improper placement, shift in screw or even breakage are not rare.

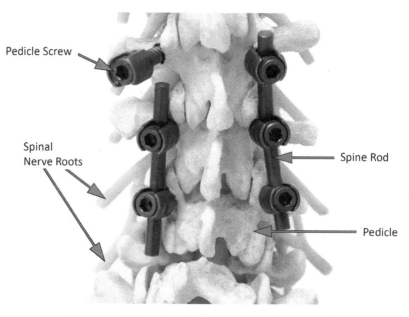

Pedicle Screw

Spinal
Nerve Roots

Spine Rod

Pedicle

Spine model with pedicle screws and spinal rods
(Note close proximity of pedicle screws to nerve roots.)

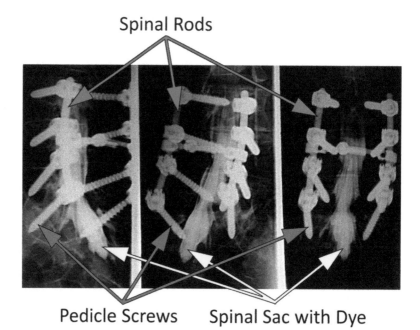

Spinal Rods

Pedicle Screws Spinal Sac with Dye

Horrifying example (actual patient x-ray) of what could happen
to your back from a knife-happy spine surgeon

These are all different types of hardware to stabilize a surgically treated spine. During a fusion procedure, bone graft fragments, spine cages and spinal hardware are combined for additional stability of the spine.

The pedicle screws can cause pain in and of themselves. They must be placed with extreme precision and if placed incorrectly, they can be touching a spinal nerve root. The fusion can fail to heal completely, therefore the spine is not as stable as it should be. All of these factors combined can result in additional pain or worsening of existing pain. Taking the pedicle screws out does not always result in clearing the pain—plus it requires another back surgery—increasing your complication rate.

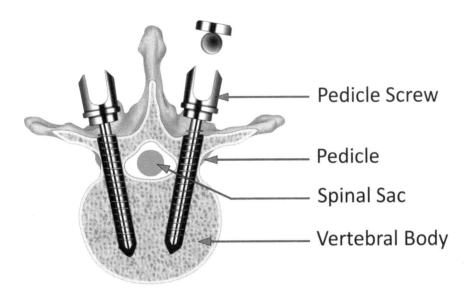

Pedicle Screw

Pedicle

Spinal Sac

Vertebral Body

Properly placed pedicle screws for spine stabilization

Anesthesia Complications

To have back surgery, or many other surgeries, you need to have general anesthesia. General anesthesia opens an entirely different Pandora's Box of potential complications. These might include heart trouble (irregular heartbeats), lung problems, bronchitis or worse: pneumonia, stroke, blood clots, and even death. Fortunately, with modern day general anesthesia, the risk of complications is low unless you are a smoker or have pre-existing heart, lung, or vascular disease.

Narcotic Addiction—a National Epidemic

Narcotic addiction is another frequent unintentional consequence following spine and other surgeries. Many patients are taking opioid pain killers prior to surgery. After the surgery is over, pain continues or is worse, so the patient is given more and even stronger narcotics to control pain. It is a vicious cycle: pain persists and worsens, and multiple addictive opioids are taken. As the effects of lower potency narcotics wear off, stronger pain killers are needed. This is how patients end up taking Oxycontin, oxycodone, hydromorphone (Dilaudid), morphine derivatives, hydrocodone, Fentanyl and other powerful, highly addictive and potentially lethal narcotics.

Chronic pain associated with failed back surgery causes anxiety. Now you are taking Xanax® (alprazolam). Alprazolam is the crack cocaine of medicine. It is extremely addictive but in an insidious way. You may not realize you are addicted until you try to stop taking this. Your body and brain become addicted to these drugs and you cannot get off of them, even if you want to (many do not). Your body becomes used to the effect of narcotics and therefore "craves" the feeling of being on these pain killers and/or alprazolam (Xanax®). Unfortunately, the body still craves the narcotic even after it stops masking pain as well and triggers other symptoms of illness.

The combination of persistent pain and being on long term, relatively high-dose narcotics, is a downward lifestyle spiral, ultimately leading to disability and a miserable quality of life. Memory loss, sedation, and generally feeling ill are documented side effects of being on narcotic therapy. Much of all of the above could have been avoided, had the person not had unnecessary back or neck surgery in the first place. Add repeated spinal surgeries to this mix and the complication rate, as well as risk for narcotic addiction and disability goes up astronomically. Unfortunately so does the rate of overdose and death.

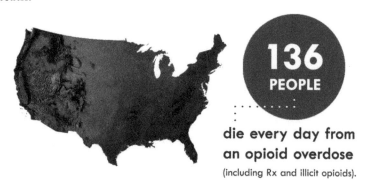

136 PEOPLE

die every day from an opioid overdose
(including Rx and illicit opioids).

Opioid Narcotics Are a Major Cause of Death

Opioids—prescription and illicit—are the main cause of drug overdose deaths in the US. Opioids were involved in over 70,000 deaths in 2017, and opioid overdoses have increased 800% since 1999. Drug overdose death rates in the United States have more than quadrupled since 1990 and have never been higher.

There is currently a steadily growing, deadly epidemic of prescription painkiller abuse. Nearly three out of four prescription drug overdoses are caused by prescription opioid painkillers. These drugs were involved in over 72,000 overdose deaths in 2017, more than cocaine and heroin combined.[67] The misuse and abuse of prescription painkillers was responsible for over one million emergency department visits in 2017. The CDC estimates that in 2017, **192 Americans died every day** from opioid overdose—half of these are due to prescription narcotics.

Three Waves of the Rise in Opioid Overdose Deaths

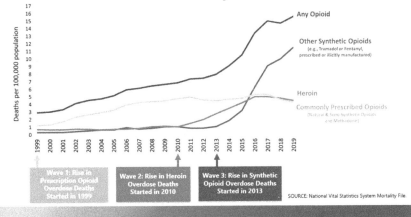

SOURCE: National Vital Statistics System Mortality File.

It is estimated that 15% of the public is genetically predisposed to opioid addiction after taking narcotic pain killers. From 2000 to 2017, more than half a million people died from drug overdoses. (See current CDC information for drug overdose data updates.) Narcotic pain killer addiction is another big risk you need to seriously consider when thinking about having spine surgery.

Opioid pain medications, following spine surgery, should not be continued for more than fifteen days.[68] A 2018 study reported treatment with opioids was not superior to treatment with non-narcotic medications for improving pain. This was also shown to be the case in an earlier study on the medication therapy for chronic lower back pain. Opioids were no more effective than anti-inflammatory agents. Conclusions in these studies did not support starting opioid therapy for moderate to severe chronic back pain or hip or knee pain.[69,70] Prescription opioid addiction can lead to heroin use. Once a patient can no longer get their prescription opioids, they still crave that narcotic high and switch to easily accessible heroin. It is a further downward spiral from there.

Reflex Sympathetic Dystrophy (RSD) or Complex Regional Pain Syndrome (CRPS)

Another painful, chronic condition known as RSD can be a complication of surgery. RSD is "a chronic pain condition that can affect any area of the body, but often affects an arm or a leg." Affected limb(s) are exquisitely sensitive to anything touching the skin. This triggers an acute wave of pain. In RSD, injured nerves can no longer control temperature, feeling, and blood flow to the affected limb and related areas. RSD is now preferentially referred to as CRPS Type 1 (RSD) where there is only a relatively minor injury and no nerve damage. CRPS Type 2 is where there is clear evidence of nerve damage.[71]

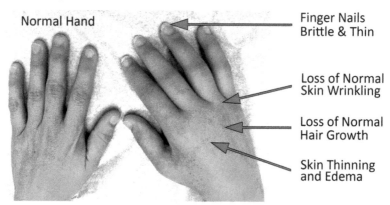

Normal Hand

Finger Nails Brittle & Thin

Loss of Normal Skin Wrinkling

Loss of Normal Hair Growth

Skin Thinning and Edema

RSD is painful, an intense burning pain that might worsen rather than improve over time. The pain can spread over an entire limb or area and even to another side of the body. Besides pain, the condition creates changes in these areas:

- Nerves
- Skin

- Thinning
- Cool skin temperature
- Mottling–blotchy, red-purplish marbling discoloration of the skin
- Swelling (edema) and sweating
- Loss of hair growth
- Finger or toe nail thinning and brittleness
- Muscle Atrophy
- Bones – accelerated osteoporosis

Other symptoms can include

- Joint pain
- Muscle spasms and eventual muscle wasting
- Swollen skin with large areas of discoloration
- Extreme sensitivity to cold
- In severe cases, contracture of the muscles leading to limited movement of the limbs

Acupuncture is one of the better palliative treatments for RSD. Although there are other symptomatic treatments, CRPS remains a serious condition for which there is no specific cure. RSD can change over time and may improve. The following pictures are of a patient who had developed RSD after undergoing neck surgery that was unnecessary:

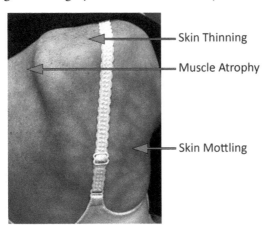

Reflex Sympathetic Dystrophy (RSD)
—skin mottling, hair loss and muscle atrophy

In summary, there are numerous, potential complications from spine surgery:

- Risks of general anesthesia
- Blood clots – pulmonary embolisms leading to death
- Sepsis – serious bacterial infections
- Spinal abscess
- Fusion failure
- Hospital acquired infections
- Neurogenic bladder
- Neurogenic erectile dysfunction–inability to orgasm
- Complex Regional Pain Syndrome Type 1 (Reflex Sympathetic Dystrophy)
- Complex Regional Pain Syndrome Type 2
- Narcotic addiction
- Never ending cycle of repeat spinal surgeries
- Spinal hardware complications including pedicle screw fracture

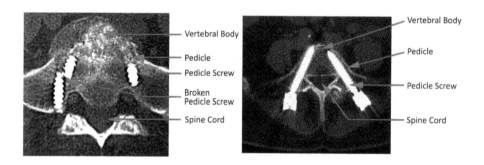

Broken pedicle screw leading to nerve root damage   *Properly placed pedicle screws for spine stabilization*

CHAPTER 7

Never-Ending Surgery Cycle

Spine surgery tends to lead to more spine surgery. You can go through surgery after surgery, without any guarantee of your pain improving. In fact, spinal surgery puts additional stress your spine, which leads to more pain. Some spine surgeons then use that new pain as justification for you to have additional surgery!

The root of the problem is the fact that persistent back pain is not an indication for back surgery, any more than persistent neck pain is an indication for neck surgery. Surgery done for the sole purpose of relieving back or neck pain is ultimately doomed to failure. This is due to the fact that the precise cause of this chronic spinal pain is not readily identified and usually multifactorial in nature.

Back surgery fails for a number of reasons. The five main reasons for Failed Back Surgery are:

1. Surgery was **never** indicated or necessary in the first place.

2. The surgical procedure performed would never have achieved the desired outcome, which is freedom from pain.

   There are only two things spine surgery can do to relieve pain: 1) decompress a nerve root, or, 2) stabilize a painful spine motion segment. That is it—nothing else.

3. Correct surgery was performed, but did not get the intended result.

4. Poor surgical technique.

5. Spinal hardware including screws, rods, plates, cages, and artificial discs creating an additional source for pain.

Is Spine Surgery Beneficial to Anyone?

Why are these unnecessary procedures so often done, if they do not help patients? As in many areas of life, the reason lies in the familiar answer, "follow the money." Procedures performed primarily for reasons of secondary gain such as Workers' Compensation, automobile accident insurance, or other liability legal claims are significant predictors of poor outcomes. Individuals who undergo spine surgery for the purpose of settling a claim typically end up with chronic neck and/or back pain. They are the losers in this ongoing saga. Tragically, the only people who win are the surgeons, pain doctors, pharmaceutical companies, and the lawyers.

I have heard that the *need* for spine surgery is increasing, have you? Would you really believe that the incidence of medically justifiable, surgically treatable spine disease is going to triple in the next five years? Not only would this be considered a national epidemic, but also a major public health crisis. "Better procedures," "smaller incisions," and "new technology in spine hardware" are just a few of the cited reasons used to justify an exponential increase in the *need* for spine surgery.[72] None of these would lead to an *increase in the need* for spine surgery. This, however, is what the spine surgery industry would have you believe. It is like the spine surgery industry is marketing to you "prime waterfront property" which really turns out to be swamp land. Yes this con is that unethical, in my opinion.

The trend toward doing more and more spine surgery is disturbing! It has been reported that so-called need for "Spine Care" (translation: "spine surgery") will dramatically rise over the next decade. Reasons cited for this upsurge include increases in spinal injuries, obesity, aging population, more athletic injuries, and better spine surgery techniques and instrumentation.[73]

This reminds me of a story where a dentist was accused of unnecessarily pulling teeth, even healthy ones, as his panacea cure for any ailment in someone's mouth. "People have higher-sugar diets, these days," he said. "One rotting tooth leads to more," he justified. Turned out that it was more profitable for him to sell as many denture sets as possible and also fire three of his four hygienists. Lower overhead, more profit. The difference here is, at least the dentist solved the patient's problem in one radical manner, and didn't simply give them an aspirin and bill. There are Codes of Ethics and that is what my message is in this book: medical professionals (including spine surgeons) should put ethics and sound medical recommendations first.

Patients (like those suffering with severe neck or back pain) should be aware that, in fact, not all medical professionals are doing that.

Further reports suggest that since more children and teens are playing sports and requiring repetitive physical training, a significant growth in the spine care (i.e., spine surgery) market will occur. Conversely, the same report acknowledges the rate of obesity in the US is continuously rising. An increase of the obesity epidemic leads to further spine stress, spinal degeneration, and "spinal problems." This will allegedly cause a "spur [in] spinal growth" (i.e. spine surgery) in the upcoming years.[74]

This claim of more spinal disease without any proof to justify more invasive spine procedures is ludicrous. This includes "Minimally Invasive Spine Surgery," something we affectionately refer to as "MIS" because that is what happens the surgeons "miss" the goal of you being able to live pain free. Supposedly, as the population ages, "we can expect an influx of spinal problems." Reports suggest that the aging population is expected to help fuel the spinal market. Fuel *what*? More spine surgery? Really!? Just because we are all getting older and over 85% of us will have some episode of back pain in our lives, does not justify a rampant increase in the *need* for more spine surgery. Just like an aging population may result in more subscriptions to *Senior Living Magazine* being sold, but this does not prove an increase in the *need* for that particular magazine. Again, **more** spine surgery **does not mean better** healthcare or better results. Actually the reverse is true. The end result of more (unnecessary) spine surgery is just more failed back pain surgery victims.

Regarding the trends with children and sports injuries which are cited to support an increase in the need for spine surgery, which is it—there is going to be more obesity or, there is going to be more sports-related need? While obesity is certainly becoming a national health problem, it is not clear that more children nationwide are competing in sports. The proposition of having obesity and more children exercising is a contradiction in and of itself. Sports injuries, obesity, and aging do not necessarily result in an escalating need for more spine surgery.

Finally, a purported increase in spine surgery over the next decade would be "better implants." Better spine implants? So what! Just because technology allows us to make allegedly better spine hardware is again no scientific or medical proof for increasing the already too high annual number of spine surgeries performed.[75] This is the disturbing trend of using statistics to justify an end. (Just because today's engineers can now build a car that can reach speeds of over 300 mph and drive itself does not mean more and more people should therefore trade in their Honda to get one.)

The logic is flawed: True–True–Unrelated. A good analogy would be this: over the past 5 years, more people are watching more television. Over the past 5 years, there has been increasing destruction of the rain forest. Therefore, it stands to reason that more people watching television causes accelerated rain forest destruction. Just because the two issues are occurring at the same time does not mean they have anything to do with one another.

Minimally Invasive Spine Surgery (MIS) is projected to rise at an annual growth rate of about eight percent through 2025. Amazing! That would mean that by some magical process, the incidence of true, operable spine disease is **mysteriously going to increase by eight percent every year** through 2025. This is Alice-in-Wonderland thinking. The fact of the matter is that justifiable, objective, surgically treatable spine disease occurrence has remained stable over the past 20 years.[76]

What has increased is the *lack* of detailed patient physical examinations, close review of MRI spine results, and correlating them directly with the objective neurological deficits the patient may (or may not) have. If the exam is normal and shows no evidence of neurological compromise, it is not really possible to justify any spine surgery. It is at this exact moment where there is a *lack of critical thinking* by the doctor who makes the recommendation for spine surgery. Unfortunately, being driven by the medical hardware industry and just plain greed, spine surgery is on the ever rising upswing.

The robotic spine surgery industry is beginning to play a role in minimally invasive spine surgery (MIS). These advanced computer software systems reportedly allow the robotic machines to make extremely precise movements. *Big deal!* If spine surgery was never indicated in the first place, it does not matter how precise the cut is made or how quick the healing time— it should have never been made at all. The worldwide spine surgery robotics market was valued at $26 *Million* in 2017 and is expected to reach about $3 BILLION by 2022. This is based on the fact that, in the United States, over 1.5 million spinal operations are performed annually, while the worldwide number is approximately 5 million. This means that nearly one third of all spine surgeries are performed in only one country, the United States, whose population accounts for only 4% of the world population.[77]

You know, I had a printer on my desk one time that could not print a decent, clear, black-ink document page no matter what I tried (including buying expensive, heavy, printer paper and new brand-name ink cartridges). Every white sheet had at least one smudge or line of text that was blurred. Now imagine that I take it in to a computer and printer tech support center and tell them of my "pain" and their answer is, "You should buy this expensive plug-in for the printer which makes it print 10 times faster." *So I can waste ten times as much expensive paper and ink every day? How does this help solve my problem?* "Your printer is an older model. You can get this leading-edge technology that will improve your printing speed and save you tons of time." The similarity is that when a doctor you go to for a solution is only focused on selling you new spine surgery technology *when it won't solve your problem,* that doctor's license should go in the shredder along with all my fuzzy-printed rejects.

In this country, over 30 million people suffer from chronic back pain.[78] The surgical industry mentality is that there is a potential for performing more spine surgery if the phenomenal accuracy and magical pain relief can be falsely promised due to better surgery from robots. This disingenuous propaganda for spinal surgery is the reason there are so many Americans living with Failed Back Syndrome and chronic pain—spine surgery would have never made them better, robotic, laser, endoscopic surgery, MIS, fusion or any other operation.[79]

A newer, non-surgical pain intervention procedure has been developed. This treatment is for spinal stenosis, narrowing of the lower back spinal canal. Similar to other medieval practices (circa 900 A.D), two large trocars, a tool also used for embalming, are inserted into the lower back spine. Then metal spacers are inserted and used as jacks or shims to separate and hold the spine vertebrae apart. The problem with this questionable procedure is that it does not treat the actual spinal stenosis. The problem, spinal stenosis, *is still there* and will continue to worsen. Meanwhile, you just helped the pain specialist to pay off his new yacht.

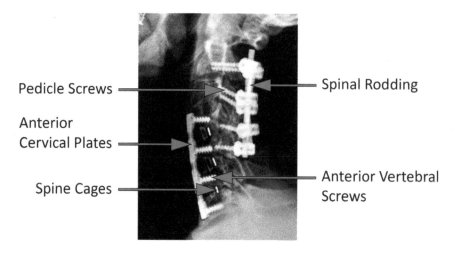

*Anterior and posterior cervical fusion with
pedicle screws, spinal rods and fusion cages*

It is a well-documented fact that individuals suffering from chronic lower back pain do not improve with new or additional back surgery. Why? The cause of chronic lower back pain is a poorly defined problem with no identifiable cause. This problem does grow every year.[80] The cause of chronic lower back pain is complex and multifactorial, most of the time having nothing to do with spine disorders. In the spine surgery world, minimally invasive spine surgery (MIS) is projected to grow 9 percent per year from 2016-2022. To translate that into numbers, that is a growth in expenditure of medical dollars from $14 billion in 2016 to almost $23 billion in 2022. That is the annual spending just for minimally invasive back surgery alone! There is no reason to believe that the annual increase will ever stop, without intervention from Medicare and insurance companies insisting on effective conservative care instead of high cost, ineffective surgery.

Fortunately, an increasing number of healthcare providers and some health insurers are beginning to realize there is a better and more effective way to manage low back pain other than surgery, considering 80% of Americans will suffer one or more episodes of back pain in their lives.[81] This more conservative treatment trend is better and has a much lower risk for complications. What they are beginning to understand is the growing body of research that shows active (hands-on) therapies and other non-surgical, non-invasive and non-drug treatment frequently is just as effective (or more so) than surgery and/or drugs.[82,83]

Lower back pain affects 8 out of 10 Americans at some point in their lives. It is one of the main reasons people go to see a doctor—a staggering 24 million visits a year. The Veterans Administration healthcare system is catching on as well. They are realizing that "conventional treatments" like surgery and other invasive procedures, may actually hinder recovery as well as promote more disability. They have realized that conservative treatment provides the best results in the majority of back and neck pain sufferers.

CASE STUDY

"Shirley" is a 75-year-old woman with lower back pain. This pain had been progressively worsening to the point where she was limited in her physical activities. The pain became sharper with lifting or walking any distance, meaning that she had trouble simply lifting a pan off the stovetop or walking out to her mailbox. A neighbor told her she should consider moving to a nursing home!

Her internist ordered an CT lumbar spine scan. Shirley did have a remote history of having prior lower back surgery at L4-5 for spinal stenosis, with good success. Her new scan showed moderate spinal stenosis at L2-3 and L3-4. Her physician was going to send her to a back surgeon for evaluation for surgery. Fortunately, she called our office and came in for non-surgical consultation.

We learned of her history of pain and treatments, and her current problems. It was clear that her back pain was isolated to the right lower back only. There was no leg pain, sciatica, or claudication. Additionally, Shirley was a high risk surgical candidate, anyway: she had known heart disease, diabetes, obesity, had atrial fibrillation, and was on prescribed blood thinners. She was treated in a very conservative manner at our clinic and recovered well. As soon as her pain significantly lessened, she became more active, lost weight, and reported she had more energy overall.

Shirley said she was glad she had not listened to the doctor who suggested seeing a back surgeon, but I don't think she realized just how fortunate she was to have made the right choice. Had she seen a back surgeon, there was a high probability that she would have had back surgery for her ASYMPTOMATIC two level mild lumbar stenosis. Not only would the surgery never have fixed the right lower back pain, it would also have put her at great risk for complications from her other medical problems, in addition to Failed Back Syndrome with crippling chronic lower back pain. A non-surgical consultation and conservative treatment was all that was needed in this case. She did well with conservative, non-surgical treatment. In the vast majority of individuals suffering from lower back pain, the MRI or CT will not give you the answer but can lead you down the path of bad outcomes.

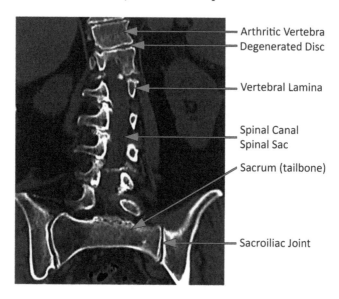

CT Lumbar spine—no stenosis
(Spinal canal wide open)

As discussed in a previous section, treatments such as narcotics—hydrocodone, oxycodone, and Fentanyl are a problem and not the cure. Awareness of opioid abuse and addiction by all healthcare professionals is improving. The Veterans Administration (VA) has reduced opioid prescribing by 25 percent from 2012 through 2016. Remember, over 70,000 Americans died in 2017 from opioid overdose.[84]

Comprehensive Review Regarding Treatment of Back Pain

Your spine is under a great deal of stress due to multiple factors including normal spine physiology, lifting, twisting, poor posture, poor body conditioning, aging, muscle atrophy, and obesity—just to name a few. All of these add up to the "perfect storm" of causing acute, recurrent and/or chronic low back pain. Unfortunately, the majority of physicians are going the opposite direction when it comes to properly managing back pain conservatively. Well-established guidelines exist for routine conservative back pain management, including use of nonsteroidal anti-inflammatory drugs

(NSAIDs) or acetaminophen with physical therapy and daily back exercise, specifically avoiding ordering early MRI imaging, oral steroids, opioid narcotics, epidural steroids or any other aggressive treatments. *Oral steroids have never been shown to be effective in management of neck or back pain.*

Aggressive treatment would include referral to a spine surgeon or pain management specialist. In the absence of neurological changes such as weakness, your back or neck pain will usually improve with conservative treatment in less than 3 months.[85]

Many general physicians, surgeons, and pain management specialists are all too quick to order more tests, particularly MRIs and give you harmful narcotic medications. Addiction, overdose, and death are serious risks with this type of back pain management. Opioid pain medication prescriptions and MRI scans ordered have more than doubled over the past ten years.[86] These disturbing numbers despite the overwhelming evidence showing that most back and neck pain will improve with conservative therapies—without any aggressive invasive treatment.

MRI scanning, narcotics, and epidural steroids would not have, in any way, changed the management and outcome of those patients who were fortunate enough to escape the surgeon's knife. With the current trends in so-called "standard" back pain treatment (MRI, steroids, narcotics), there has been *no reduction in pain or disability.* Furthermore, rates of serious complications and death are rising due to the use of invasive treatments and opioids.[87]

As a counterpoint, consider the recent history of treatment for high blood pressure, stroke and heart disease. Since the late 1970s, there has been a push for doctors to aggressively treat all individuals with high blood pressure. The medical community responded and we have seen a dramatic drop in the rate of stroke across the United States. The same is true for heart disease. Medications and advancements in cardiac procedures have had a major impact in treating and reducing the incidence of heart disease and heart attack with the associated disability and death that went along with these.

In the 1990s, new blood pressure medications such as the ACE inhibitors not only treated high blood pressure but also helped patients with heart disease as well as having a dramatic effect on stroke risk reduction. The development of coronary artery stenting has reduced the need for highly invasive heart bypass surgery. Not only is the recovery time very short for cardiac stenting—days versus weeks for bypass surgery—the complication rate is also much lower.

More testing for back and neck pain (followed by more surgery) is not the answer. If it was, we would be seeing a drop-off in second and third spine surgeries. If spine surgery really "fixed" the problem, the rate of neck and back surgeries would be going down, as we saw with reduction in stroke with aggressive treatment of high blood pressure and heart disease. With all the new spinal hardware, implants, and "new and improved" surgical techniques, everyone that has had surgery for neck or back pain should be dramatically better. At least, that is what is promised to those seeking out treatment for their neck or back pain. Unfortunately, just the opposite is happening. Spine surgery is on the ever-increasing upswing, due to more MRI scans being done and new spine implants/hardware, high spine surgery failure rate and subsequent disability that follows.

Seeing an abnormality on your CT or MRI spine scanning is common— over 70% of us have some MRI spine abnormality with virtually no symptoms at all. Unfortunately, uninformed doctors and surgeons see these imaging abnormalities and feel the need to "fix it." This is the direct cause of all too many unnecessary spine surgeries and the increasing rates of failed back and neck surgery. The simple fact is that most adult Americans are living their daily lives with MRI spine abnormalities that are not causing any symptoms at all. You know how when you go to a dermatologist for a full screening to detect possible skin cancer, the doctor sees many "abnormal" areas which may be raised or discolored, but do NOT indicate pre-cancer or melanoma, so he passes over them without reaching for a scalpel or laser. Sounds completely reasonable, doesn't it? Just because something appears differently than a perfect specimen, it does not automatically mean aggressive treatment is therefore necessary.

Psychologically, patients who see their MRI or CT scan reports start having negative thinking about themselves as well. "I can't do that anymore. I have disc bulges or disc herniations." Now they become victims of their own self-limiting MRI interpretations, believing themselves to be afflicted chronic pain patients. This is a psychological plague that can stay with them the rest of their lives. This happens, despite the fact that they are not having any symptoms related to these MRI findings. *More* testing is not necessarily better. Disc bulging never causes pain or "pinched nerves." All of this is unnecessary, self-limiting, negative thinking and behavior which ruins their quality of life. Do not let yourself become a victim of this harmful thought process. Remember, disc bulging, which does not cause pain, is only an MRI finding. In fact, most spinal changes seen on MRI or CT spine studies are chronic and degenerative in nature and cause no symptoms. They have nothing at all to do with your neck or back pain. Think of something "abnormal" on your scan as being as insignificant as a freckle your (good) dermatologist tells you not to worry about.

Over half of the patients with back pain have taken some narcotic opioid as a treatment for their pain. National guidelines have strong recommendations against the use of narcotics for treatment of both acute and chronic back pain. Side effects from opioid use can include drowsiness, confusion, memory difficulty, severe constipation, nausea, addiction and overdose resulting in death: All completely avoidable.[88,89] Treatment with opioids has not been shown to be superior to treatment with acetaminophen or nonsteroidal anti-inflammatory medications for improving pain-related function. Clearly, study results do not support initiation of narcotic opioid therapy for even severe back pain.[90]

Another review published by the JAMA looked at the summary of 20 different clinical trials, involving about 7,300 patients. The findings were that the majority of these patients reported that opioids did not provide any significant, lasting relief in those with chronic low back pain. Surgery is generally not an option in these patients as the cause for chronic low back pain is not one identifiable problem. It is a multifaceted condition for which surgery is not the answer.[91]

In the vast majority of patients with neck or back pain, the MRI findings do not correlate with their symptoms. Arthritic changes are common and are usually not the explanation for the patients' pain. Other common problems that cause chronic low back pain (and **cannot** be fixed by surgery) are strained muscles, poor posture, lack of body conditioning—just to name a few. What contributes to this? Lack of exercise, inactivity, obesity, not doing regular stretching, tight muscles, smoking, depression and negative thinking, "I have bulging and herniated discs."[92]

Depression is not often recognized as a major contributing factor to pain. Pain can amplify depression, but the converse is true as well. Recognizing the fact that you may have depression is the first step to improving your global quality of life. In the 21st century, we now have outstanding medications for treating depression. Additionally, non-drug therapies can include meditation, biofeedback assisted relaxation, yoga, and cognitive behavioral therapy. Stress reduction plays an important role in reducing pain and improving your quality of life.[93]

Do Not Just Think Twice—Avoiding Surgery Can Save Your Life

The main message here is that there are many reasons not to have back or neck surgery. Most people do not need any type of surgery for the majority of attacks of neck or back pain. Unfortunately, over half a million Americans undergo spine surgery every year. *Over half of these surgical victims will have little or no relief* of the symptoms for which surgery was promised to "fix." The initial choice to operate on a patient with chronic neck or back pain subjects them to an invasive procedure that actually never would have relieved their pain in the first place. More spine surgeries are performed per capita in the United States than any other country. Back surgery rates are 40% higher here than in any other country.[94]

For many patients with chronic back pain, the actual cause cannot be identified. If the source of pain cannot be positively identified, no type of spine surgery is going to fix it. The result of unnecessary spine surgery, particularly fusions, is continued pain, more suffering and worsening quality of life. The rate of spinal fusion surgery is increasing every year. There is no scientific evidence for what is the specific indication for fusion surgery or that this is a better procedure with improved outcomes.[95] Thousands of Americans fall victim to this epidemic fusion spine surgery plague every year.

The cost of treating back pain in the United States is $25 billion annually and is steadily rising. Factoring in Worker's Compensation claims and lost wages accounts for another $25 billion a year. Including rehabilitation costs, the global medical cost of treating neck and back pain in the United States approaches $90 billion a year.[96]

Some spinal surgeons get follow up MRI scans on patients who have continued neck or back pain after surgery. These studies are going to show additional abnormalities—evidence of prior surgery and perhaps other non-specific degenerative changes. Once again, the incorrect conclusion will be made that, "The MRI shows more spinal abnormalities, so you must need more surgery to fix the problem." The cycle of more spine surgery and chronic pain never ends.

There is no science or medical evidence to support additional surgery— just a surgeon incorrectly thinking they can "fix the pain" with more spine surgery. Add obesity, depression, smoking and other medical problems such as diabetes, heart or lung disease, and this leads to an almost 100% guarantee of surgical failure, more pain, poor quality of life and of course, disability.

The World Health Organization cites low back pain as the number one cause of life-years lost to disability worldwide.[97]

Another reason that the first spinal surgery might lead you to have more spine surgery, is that even in successful cases of surgery, the levels above and below the previously operated spinal area have compromised stability. These levels are put under more constant strain and trauma. Over the next 3-4 years after the first surgery, it is not uncommon to find problems at these additional spinal levels. This may cause you to have increasing degrees of pain and the consideration for additional spinal surgery, particularly if the first surgery is done in your forties or fifties (certainly even more so if surgery is done in your thirties.) Do not forget, however, that if you have new onset of back pain, it may and probably has nothing to do with your prior back surgery.

It is not unusual to find patients such as this who have had two or three—even more—spinal surgeries. Occasionally, these same patients have had both neck and back operations. The majority do poorly and are taking high dose narcotics for pain control. The failure rate with second spine surgery in the same area approaches 70%. Patients who have three or more spine surgeries experience greater than 90% surgical failure rate.

Remember, spinal surgery will almost never "fix" your neck or back pain, but it could lead to death! Additional surgery is not going to help most who have failed their first spine surgery, but that is precisely what is done in an unjustified attempt to relieve pain—more surgery, increased failure, more complications and adding to an already bad problem.

Surgery as a "Last Resort" is Unwise

The primary reason that spine surgery fails is this: surgery was never indicated in the first place. The specific *cause* of your back or neck pain was not specifically identified and surgery would never have "fixed" the problem, anyway. A common myth believed by the general public, and many doctors too, is that "if everything else fails, then we will try surgery." That is flawed reasoning that is not backed up with science, physiology, or medical evidence that a person with chronic pain has any specific problem that would ever be relieved with surgery. Surgery is certainly **not the cure-all** for neck or back pain, so "trying surgery as a last resort" is always a bad decision, even if you have persistent pain. Because surgery carries so many risks, as mentioned previously, using it as a last resort is not the same as simply finding out if it will help, or not. Most of the time, it is not the cure at all, but rather the poison. This is the reason that failed spine surgery is unfortunately quite common.

> Trying "surgery as a last resort"
> is always a bad decision.

CASE STUDY

David, now 79 years old, was the victim of not one, but **three unnecessary back surgeries**. His story begins at age 27, when he began having non-specific lower back pain. He worked as a truck driver and was doing daily heavy lifting and other strenuous physical activity. This went on for six years. After that, he would have flare ups of his back pain with physical activity. His pain was relieved with rest. Over the following years and decades, his low back pain became progressively more persistent, evolving into chronic, daily back pain.

Through his 40's he just lived with the pain. Like so many people, he resigned himself to chronic suffering. At no time did he have any radiating leg pain, numbness or weakness. His pain was isolated to the low back only. As it got worse, instead of better over time, he tried physical therapy, various medications, and back stretching. Nothing provided him with any lasting relief. Any movement, turning or bending would cause acute, severe worsening of his baseline back pain. By the age of 50, he could not tolerate the severe, constant back pain any longer.

He went to a doctor and an MRI lumbar spine study was performed. This showed non-specific arthritic changes, but nothing that would explain his chronic lower back pain. He continued to live with his back pain, using over-the-counter and prescription anti-inflammatory medications.

At the age of 61, he was seen by an orthopedic spine surgeon. A second lumbar spine MRI was performed. This study also showed non-specific arthritic changes in his spine. Again, no MRI findings that could explain his chronic, severe back pain. His neurological exam was normal with no findings of lumbar nerve root compromise (numbness, weakness or radiating leg pains). The surgeon recommended a two-level spinal fusion—even though there was nothing on David's two lumbar MRI scans to explain his back pain. The surgeon told him, "This should give you're the relief you are looking for."

David had his first back surgery in 2012. As we would expect, he did poorly. His lower back pain persisted with virtually no change in severity. No surprise here, as there was nothing identified on MRI scanning as a cause of the pain. The spine surgeon did this back surgery "as a treatment of last resort." A surgery doomed to failure, before it was even started. After that, David was suffering even more. Any movement such as just getting up out of bed or a chair would trigger severe back pain and spasms.

One year later, David was seen by the same spine surgeon who ordered another MRI lumbar scan. This study showed the prior surgical changes, chronic arthritic changes, and nothing new to explain his now intolerable back pain. Unfortunately David was told by the surgeon that a second back surgery "would fix the problem that was not fixed with the first back surgery." Again, as a last resort treatment, David consented to his second back surgery in 2014.

This was a 2-level fusion with pedicle screws and rods. Major back surgery. His medical bills were staggering. Tragically, even after adequate healing and extensive physical therapy, David felt no relief from constant and severe lower back pain. In fact, David's condition was worse. He had persistent, excruciating back pain and spasms. Any movement triggered waves of debilitating pain. Just standing up was a major project. At that point, he told me, "I have no quality of life. It is in the toilet."

If I had seen David initially, I would not have recommended surgery as his MRI scan did not show abnormalities that would in any way explain his pain. I would have recommended conservative treatments which have proven successful with many, many people. (By the way, one of the most effective therapeutic solutions is kinesiology—therapy that stretches and strengthens muscles back to their normal condition.)

Despite two major back surgery failures, David is now seeing another spine surgeon to consider a third back surgery. He has been advised not to have any additional spine surgery, as the *failure rate is over 90%* for a third back surgery for Failed Back Syndrome.

The Explosion of Fusions

Spinal fusions are the most overdone back surgery in the United States. Of the one half million back surgeries performed annually, about one third are fusions. The overall complication and failure rate for fusions is higher than that of any other spine surgery. Spinal fusion is **big business** and all too often, bad medicine. The need for spinal fusion is an ongoing debate but, in most cases, fusion surgery is not medically indicated.[98]

> ## Spinal fusion is big business and all too often, bad medicine.

This procedure has become "popular," but, all too frequently, spinal fusion is performed when there is no medical necessity to do so. Why do it? Follow the money. The fact it that the scientific medical community consensus is a resounding negative opinion on spinal fusion:

"For several low back disorders, no advantage has been demonstrated for fusion over surgery without fusion, and complications are common."[99,100]

The Agency for Health Care Policy and Research was tasked to determine how to spend Medicare dollars most effectively, and in 1994 published a report on acute back pain management.[101] The conclusion that spinal fusion surgery showed no advantage over standard spine surgery did not sit well with the spinal surgery industry. Political Action Lobbyists pressured Congress to reduce Medicare's research budget by a massive 21%. Medicare's ex- Chief Medical Officer Sean Tunis stated:

"The larger damage was the message sent by Congress: '**If you get too close to actually changing how clinical or reimbursement decisions are made, Congress is going to slap you down.** I think everyone took a lesson from that."[102]

Then it was off to the races for the multi-billion dollar spine industry to do spine fusion surgeries. In a 20-year period, spinal fusion surgeries went from 50,000 to almost a half million per year in the United States. This number continues to grow exponentially every year. This represents one spinal fusion for every 600 Americans, four times higher than most other countries. To put it another way, the rate of spine surgery is 40% higher in the US than any other country.[103] Are we seriously to believe that Americans have four times the amount of surgically treatable spine disease than the rest of the world?

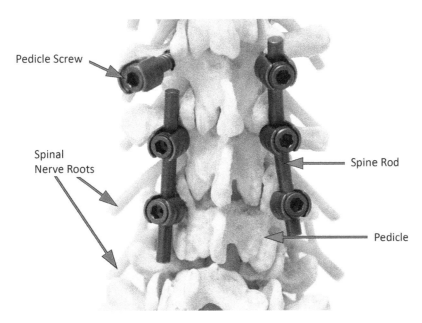

Multiple level fusion using pedicle screws and spine rods

One spine condition that is frequently treated with fusion surgery is degenerative spine disc disease, commonly known as *spinal arthritis*. Study after study has resoundingly shown no benefit for treatment of spinal arthritis with fusion surgery. Of numerous studies published, only one showed questionable benefit, but it was funded by a spinal fusion hardware company. Medicare's panel understandably dismissed the results from the spine hardware company funded study and recommended that spinal fusion *NOT* be used to treat degenerative disc disease. However, because of political pressure, the panel's recommendations were not adopted, and Medicare still pays for this unnecessary, ineffective, often harmful, and always expensive procedure.

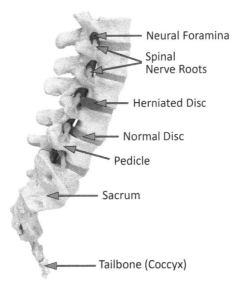

Lumbar spine model showing herniated disc

To illustrate the point of why spine surgery is not the great panacea for back pain, a retrospective study looked at 1450 individuals with chronic lower back pain. Half of the patients had lumbar fusion back surgery and the other half received conservative, non-surgical therapy for similar symptoms. At the end of two years, post-injury, a comparison showed that the surgically treated group was doing much worse than the conservatively treated group. Of those treated with fusion back surgery, only one-out-of-four went back to work compared to two out of three treated conservatively (without surgery).[104] Translated, that indicates **back fusion surgery has a 75% failure rate**.

Also, the death rate was about 50% higher in the surgically treated group. Narcotic usage was much higher as well—three out of four were using opioid pain killers at two years post-surgery. Of the surgically treated patients, one third had significant post-surgical complications. Repeat surgery was done in one out of three who failed their first surgery. The conclusion of this report was that lumbar fusion for the diagnoses of disc degeneration, disc herniation, and/or radiculopathy in a Workers' Compensation setting is associated with significant increase in disability (seven times greater following surgery), opiate use, prolonged work loss, poor chance of returning to work and lastly more disability.[105] An interesting fact came out of this study: Smoking, having legal representation and litigation are negative predictors of a favorable outcome and returning to work.[106] Individuals without legal representation were three times more likely to return to work.

Five billion dollars, every year. In America, the annual cost for spinal fusion hardware alone is more than $5 billion, double what the rest of the entire world spends combined. Spine neurosurgeons average $2,000,000 in wages per year. Over $200,000,000 was spent in 2011 for unnecessary spinal fusion procedures. These numbers just keep increasing every year and are expected to double within 10 years.

Medical experts agree that unless there is spinal deformity or instability, spinal fusion should not be performed for cases of disc degeneration (arthritis), disc herniation, or stenosis. Nevertheless, in a recent 10-year period, the number of spinal fusions in Florida alone increased by 500%. This is one of the most common causes of Failed Back Surgery resulting in chronic neck or back pain and opioid prescriptions.

"Florida has become the main source in America for prescription drugs diverted for illicit use. In 2009, for example, 98 of the top 100 oxycodone prescribers in the nation were in Florida. DEA evidence revealed that Florida prescribers wrote prescriptions for 19 million doses of oxycodone."[107] CDC data showed that over 70,000 Americans died in 2017 due to opioid overdose in that year alone.[108]

Voicing his criticism regarding spinal fusions, nationally recognized authority on back pain management, Richard Deyo, MD, was quoted as saying: "My hunch is that half of the spinal fusions in the U.S. are unnecessary"[109] Back surgery isn't like getting a haircut. There can be major complications…People who have spinal fusion surgery often feel better, just as people who go to the YMCA often feel better. The truth of the matter is that most people improve eventually on their own."[110]

Dr. Deyo also presented an abstract that noted that even with new fusion technology surgery, the rate of repeat surgery was no lower than the rates after standard decompression alone. Dr. Deyo also published a report on the comprehensive overview of lower back pain. In this review, it is clear that low back pain is common and most Americans will experience one or more episodes of back pain in their lifetime. Conservative treatment and other non-surgical treatment provided the best outcome, in most cases.[111]

Trends and Variations in the Use of Spine Surgery

The highest rate of back surgery is in the United States. More back surgeries, including discectomies, laminectomies and spinal fusions, are done here annually, with a steady increase in numbers of procedures performed every year. The reason for this includes new procedures, new types of spine hardware, and robotic back surgery.

Dr. Deyo further elaborated on the questionable choices of different back surgery techniques performed for the same type of spinal problem. If several patients have the same spinal problem, then there should be a consensus on a specific surgical technique to treat that spine disorder. Quite the opposite is the case in the US. Dr. Deyo's research showed that there was a widespread variation in spinal fusion surgeries across the country. If there was a clear medical agreement on when spinal fusions should be performed, the rates of spinal fusion surgery should be consistent throughout the country. Instead, we find a wide variation in the numbers of spinal fusion procedures done across the country.[112] The upshot of all this is that the rates of doing spinal fusions for treatment of back pain have more than tripled over the past 25 years. With the accelerating rate of new spine surgery techniques, more back surgeries are being performed. **Despite new technologies, rates of repeat** back surgery after spinal fusion were no lower than the rates after standard spine decompression surgery alone.[113]

The same is true for another new cervical spine surgical procedure known as Artificial Disc Replacement (ADR). Published studies have shown that as compared to the "standard" cervical decompression surgery (anterior discectomy cervical fusion, ACDF), **the reoperation rate for ADR is significantly higher.**[114]

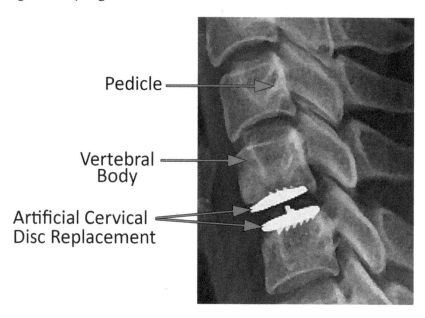

Pedicle

Vertebral Body

Artificial Cervical Disc Replacement

Artificial disc replacement in the neck – cervical spine

Overtreating Chronic Back Pain: Time to Back Off?

Chronic back pain is among the most common patient complaints. Its prevalence and impact have spawned a rapidly expanding range of tests and treatments. Some of these have become widely used for indications that are not well validated, leading to uncertainty about efficacy and safety, increasing complication rates, and marketing abuses. Recent studies document a 629% increase in Medicare expenditures for epidural steroid injections; a 423% increase in expenditures for opioids for back pain; a 307% increase in the number of lumbar magnetic resonance images among Medicare beneficiaries; and a 220% increase in spinal fusion surgery rates.

The limited studies available suggest that these increases have not been accompanied by population-level improvements in patient outcomes or disability rates. We suggest a need for a better understanding of the basic science of pain mechanisms, more rigorous and independent trials of many treatments, a stronger regulatory stance toward approval and post-marketing surveillance of new drugs and devices for chronic pain, and a chronic disease model for managing chronic back pain.[115]

Considering that disc decompression techniques cost about $12,000 with reasonably good success rate versus $80,000 for spinal fusion with overall lower rates of success. It is obvious why a spine surgeon would recommend a more expensive procedure even though it has a lower success rate.

Microdiscectomies

A note about microdiscectomy spine surgery: while this procedure is promoted as less invasive with shortened recovery time, the re-operation rate is significantly higher than standard Minimally Invasive Spine Surgery. Often, the victim of a failed microdiscectomy procedure is then subjected to a second, traditional spine surgery or even worse, spinal fusion. The outcomes of many second back surgeries are frequently poor.

Recovery: Time-Consuming and Costly

Recovery from spine surgery is not a minor matter. With a straightforward lumbar or cervical disc removal and laminectomy (Minimally Invasive Spine Surgery), full recovery may be 8 weeks. Surgical healing time after a fusion is 10-12 weeks. Many people do not realize that **no fusion happens at the time of surgery**—clinically significant spine fusion does not even begin until six months post-surgery. A fusion procedure, particularly at multiple levels, may take well over a year. In a spinal fusion surgery, the spine does not always fuse, resulting in Failed Back Surgery.[116]

Healthy, timely recovery is based on the fact that you are generally in good health. Conditions that drastically compromise healing include smoking, diabetes, heart or lung disease, obesity, and daily alcohol use, just to name a few.

During this recovery time, patients may be sent for varying courses of physical therapy and rehabilitation. This process is time consuming, laborious and expensive. The time consuming and expensive part comes from missed time off work, missing school and not being able to participate in family activities. Additionally, spine fusion surgeries have a high rate of the spine not "fusing" – almost 1 out of 5 incidence. This leads to more spine instability, pain, additional spine surgery and even longer recovery time. Many such patients never recover. **Important consideration**: right or wrong, spine surgery is not reversible.

Some spine surgeons may actually believe that the surgery they are doing for neck or back pain will benefit you. This is particularly true for spine centers that offer "proprietary spine surgery." They base this on their own personal observations (clearly biased) or on anecdotal, observational published studies—not rigorously scientific or medically accurate. The general belief of spine surgeons that spine surgery will be effective and successful for low back pain is not supported by the bulk of the published, well-conducted clinical trials. The most credible trials regarding outcomes of spine surgery show that only a small percentage of patients do well (less than 40%).[117] Most patients continue to have lasting pain, sometimes more severe than before their surgery.

If the spine surgeon community believes that their outcomes are better than what the current, controlled clinical trial studies show, they should publish their results for all the community and other clinicians to review. Beware of what they promise you on their "million dollar" websites. In the absence of objective, verifiable information, the actual benefits from neck or back surgery must be seriously questioned.[118]

Since the benefits of spine surgery are small, very specific and careful patient selection is absolutely essential for good outcomes. You need to be informed of the specific problem for which spine surgery is proposed, the surgical procedure being used, expected outcome, potential risks, and non-surgical alternatives in order that you may make an informed decision as to proceed with spinal surgery or not. The surgical community has never defined what is the "critically selected patient" criteria for successful spine surgery – tested by evidence-based medicine studies.[119]

Based on what hundreds of patients have told me, I have concluded that if you went to five different spine surgeons with your spine MRI scan, you will probably receive five different opinions on what treatment you need—from "it's not a surgically treatable problem" to "you need a three-level laminectomy with rodding, cage and fusion." Who's right? Most likely the one that told you not to have surgery.

In conclusion, spinal fusion should not be proposed as a standard treatment for chronic low back pain, or any back pain, for that matter. The cause of nonspecific spinal pain is complex and chronic low back pain should not be regarded as a specific diagnosis, but rather a complex collection of symptoms in affected patients with different stages of pain, impairment and disability. Patients with chronic back pain (CLBP) should be evaluated in a multidisciplinary setting, not involving surgery or invasive procedures, according to the biopsychosocial model, which aims to identify underlying psychosocial factors as well as biological (physical) factors.

Treatment should occur in a stepwise fashion, starting with the least invasive, generally conservative treatment. The recommended 21st century comprehensive treatment approach to CLBP, is emphasis on self-management and enabling patients to take active participation in the treatment of their back pain, in order to prevent long-term disability and chronicity.[120,121] This information comes as little comfort for the majority of post-spine surgery patients who have already been permanently victimized from not doing well, who suffer complications, habituated to narcotics or who are rendered worse after spine surgery.

Other Considerations Regarding Your Spine Health

Consequences of Unnecessary Spinal Surgery: Failed Back Syndrome

Failed Back Syndrome, or Post-Laminectomy Syndrome, is the term given to patients who have had spine surgery, but continue to have pain or worsening of their pain. As stated previously, the root of the problem is the fact that back pain is not an indication for back surgery, any more than neck pain is an indication for neck surgery.

Surgery done for the sole purpose of relieving isolated back or neck pain is going to lead to more pain. Even worse, the scarring created as a natural result of surgery can lead to additional pain that can be even more difficult to treat. All too many spinal surgeons make the false assumption that if a patient still has back pain, and there is an MRI abnormality, this is the cause of their pain and more surgery is necessary.

> MRI evaluation in adults with no symptoms showed herniated discs in 7 out of 10 people.

In actuality, just the opposite is true. Most causes of back or neck pain cannot be identified with MRI, CT or any other imaging—before or after spine surgery. If you see a spine surgeon, you are going to get a surgical opinion. This very commonly includes a surgery recommendation. If you see a pain management specialist they are going to recommend epidural steroids, facet nerve blocks, radio frequency ablation and narcotic pain killers, indefinitely. The underlying cause of your pain will never be treated but rather just the symptoms. The better option is to see a neurologist or physical medicine specialist for conservative back and neck pain treatment and management. Even then, see a non-surgical specialist who **specializes** in the non-surgical treatment of neck or back pain.

Failed Back Syndrome (FBS) has many different causes. Some of these include operating at the wrong level, failure to remove the entire herniated disc fragment, nerve damage, trauma to the exiting nerve root, continued pressure on the nerve root, scar tissue and chronic inflammatory changes at the site of surgery known as arachnoiditis, an incurable disease.[122] There is no scientifically-based, proven treatment to prevent, reverse or cure arachnoiditis. Arachnoiditis treatment, at best, is palliative pain control.[123]

Back surgery typically involves removing some of the boney part of the spine. This can result in spinal instability associated with excessive movement at the site of surgery. This causes additional spinal trauma and pain. Predisposing factors to FBS include smoking, diabetes, obesity, vascular disease (hardening of the arteries), poor pre-surgical physical conditioning or other diseases that predispose to a weak immune system (e.g. rheumatoid, lupus, sarcoidosis, depression, alcohol abuse). Other poor prognostic factors include neck or back pain from auto accidents, concurrent litigation or workers' compensation claims.[124]

FBS symptoms include persistent dull back pain, which can vary in intensity. At times, you may have sharp back pains that may radiate down one or both legs. You can also have abnormal painful leg numbness. In almost all cases of failed back syndrome, more surgery is the worst thing that can be done, as this only compounds an already difficult painful condition. Additionally, surgery does not treat the underlying core muscle weakness, muscle tightness and loss of flexibility. All of these latter components must be treated and resolved to have a great outcome.

There are 80,000 new cases of failed back surgery every year in the United States. Approximately 20% of these cases will undergo a second spine surgery. With repeated back surgery the success rates plummet to 30%, 15% and finally 5% with each successive second, third and fourth spine surgeries. [125] Why would you have even a second spine surgery if you knew that there is a 70% probability that that surgery would fail.[121] Did your spine surgeon tell you that? If driving, golfing or skiing had those kind of odds for permanent injury, you would probably not be driving, golfing or skiing anymore.

Of those that have spinal fusions, over half will never return to work. Workers' compensation patients have the poorest overall outcomes for all spine surgery.[126,127] Spinal fusions have a much higher rate of failure than other types of spine surgery.[128] It is estimated that there are 2-3 million Americans suffering from Failed Back Syndrome, with that number growing every year. Prevention of FBSS is the key.[129]

"The doctor of the future will give no medicine, but will instruct his patients in care of the human frame, in diet, and in the cause and prevention of disease."

—Thomas Edison

CHAPTER 8

What Are The Conditions That May Require Back Surgery?

The reasons to have back or neck surgery are few. **All criteria for successful spinal surgery must be met prior to considering or undergoing spine surgery.**

1. Spinal stenosis in the lower back of sufficient degree to cause claudication (pain in the legs with walking any distance that clears promptly with rest).

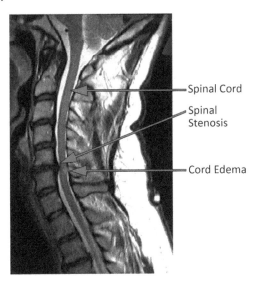

Spinal Cord

Spinal Stenosis

Cord Edema

2. Spinal stenosis in the cervical spine of less than 9 mm associated with even slight spinal cord deformity. The risk of severe spinal cord damage in the neck is high if combined with traumatic injuries to the neck, such as whiplash trauma.

3. Disc herniations that are clearly causing nerve root compression and these findings correlate exactly with the patient's complaints of pain, numbness and/or weakness and corresponding abnormal findings on neurological exam. Conservative therapy should always be tried first.

4. Stenosis of the neural foramen (the small openings where the nerve roots exit the boney spine). If a patient has definite symptoms of this condition, he/she should have numbness, pain and weakness in the distribution of the compressed nerve. For example, a right C6 nerve root compression will not cause left arm pain or weakness. Symptoms of a right C6 nerve root compression include numbness down the arm into the thumb and along the thumb side of the forearm, biceps pain and/or weakness. There may not be any neck pain at all.

5. Bulging discs ARE NEVER a sufficient reason to justify neck or back surgery.

6. Stabilize a painful spine joint segment – Stage 2, 3 or 4 spondylolisthesis.

7. Additional reason to have spine surgery includes other more serious problems such as tumors, cancer or fractures of the spine. These conditions are beyond the scope of this book.

Why Do I Have Back Or Neck Pain?
What Is The Treatment For It?

Treatment of Lower Back and Neck Pain–Without Surgery

Fortunately, for you, there are several highly effective non-surgical, non-narcotic back pain treatment options. This applies if you have not had surgery or for those with post-surgical neck or back pain. The main treatment for back and neck pain is general body conditioning, stretching, core conditioning, keeping your body weight under control and regular exercise. For you to have good neck and back health, daily neck/back exercise and stretching is required. These are simple exercises that, once learned, take you only a few minutes a day. These exercises will keep your neck/back muscles stretched out, balanced and in good condition. Adding some abdomen muscle strengthening on a regular basis will add to your continued back health.

EXERCISES TO RELIEVE BACK PAIN

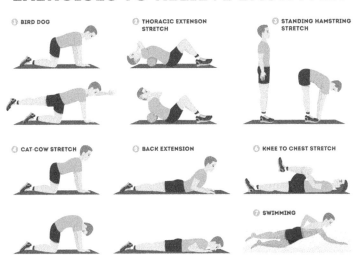

STRETCH FOR NECK AND SHOULDER PAIN

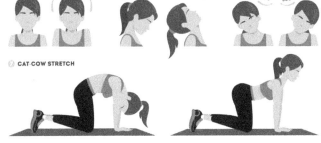

When you notice pain and discomfort in your neck or back, it is most often due to soft tissue tightness and inflammation. This is not a spinal problem, but is rather in the muscles and fascia surrounding your spine. Simple, but specific, soft tissue injections (NOT epidural steroids or trigger point injections) can provide dramatic relief, in combination with exercise and therapy. If your neck or back pain persists, manual, hands-on physical therapy can be helpful.

Effective Non-surgical Treatment of Neck and Back Pain

The vast majority of neck and back pain is not due to any problems with the spine, spinal cord or spinal nerve roots. The underlying cause of pain is due to soft tissue pain. Soft tissue pain includes pain from muscles, ligaments, tendons and fascia. Fascia is the covering that surrounds all muscles for strengthening and protection. Fascia also wraps every organ and blood vessel in the body. It has multiple functions, which we are still discovering.[130] Fascia contains a high number of nerve pain fibers. Inflammation of the fascia is frequently what is causing much of your neck, back, arm, or leg pains. Just like muscles, fascia can become tight, irritated and painful.

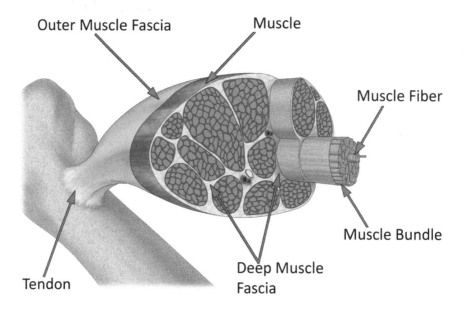

Fascia is found extensively throughout all muscles

One of the most significant causes for underlying pain is muscle imbalances in the neck, shoulder girdle, pelvic girdle, hips, legs, and lower back. Muscle imbalances lead to weakness in certain muscles with other muscles overcompensating for this weakness. This results in the supporting muscles becoming overused, tight and painful. This is vicious pain-spasm cycle that leads to weakness and atrophy of the weaker muscles.

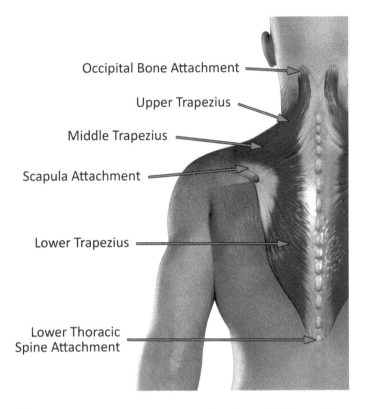

Occipital Bone Attachment

Upper Trapezius

Middle Trapezius

Scapula Attachment

Lower Trapezius

Lower Thoracic
Spine Attachment

The massive trapezius muscle attaches from the base of the skull and shoulder blade down to the mid-lower back

These muscles are the support system for the hip, pelvis and lower back. Your body can compensate for the weaker muscles by overusing and stressing out the stronger muscles. This results in painful tightness, spasm and trigger points in various lower back, buttocks and hip/leg muscles.

Compensating for muscle imbalance causes you to have imbalances in your gait. Changing from a more natural way of walking can temporarily give a slight reprieve from pain, but gait imbalances result in shortened gait, loss of flexibility, tightness, and more pain. Over a period of time, you are not aware this is occurring until you exceed your body's limit and ability to compensate for the weak muscles. The result is painful muscle and fascia spasm with tissue inflammation. This is your first noticeable symptom of hip, back and/or leg pain. Still, this has nothing to do with the spine, spinal nerves, or sciatic nerve. And NONE of these causes of pain can be seen on MRI or CT scanning.

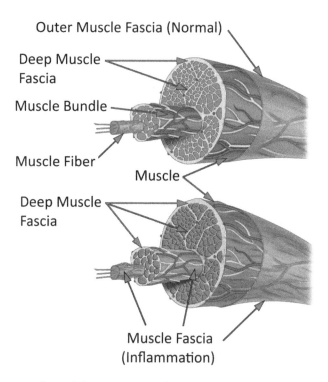

Outer Muscle Fascia (Normal)

Deep Muscle Fascia

Muscle Bundle

Muscle Fiber

Muscle

Deep Muscle Fascia

Muscle Fascia (Inflammation)

Inflamed fascia surrounding muscles causes pain

What Does All This Mean?

It means that in most cases, your neck, lower back, hip, buttocks and leg pain are due to muscle tightness with weakness, muscle strength imbalance, loss of flexibility all resulting in pain. This also includes the muscles and tendons making up the hip and shoulder girdles. None of these problems can be diagnosed with MRI, CT, or any other diagnostic test. Diagnosis is 100% dependent on a detailed hands-on physical examination, by qualified healthcare providers, or specialized therapists. Routine exams by your primary care doctor, orthopedic surgeon, neurosurgeon, or physical therapist most likely will not find these problems. A highly trained physical therapist, exercise physiologist, kinesiologist or osteopathic physician can diagnose these soft tissue problems easily and recommend appropriate corrective therapy.

Routine physical therapy—hot/cold packs, ultrasound, electrical stimulation, and/or cold laser therapy—has not been shown to be effective and will have virtually no healing effect to solve the underlying problem. These are all treatments for symptoms only with temporary relief at best, but does not correct the underlying cause.

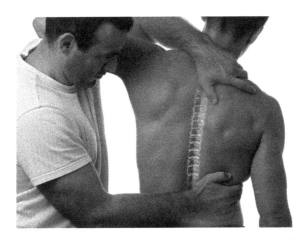

Corrective manual therapy for back muscles and fascia

The only treatment for these muscle imbalances is corrective, hands-on therapy. Your qualified therapist first needs to identify both the weak, tight and overused muscles. Then the tight, overused muscles and fascia will need to be actively stretched and lengthened to create a balance reset followed by strengthening of the weaker muscles to restore the normal, physiological balance in the neck, shoulder girdle, lower back, hip, pelvic and leg muscles.

The end game is an overall restoration of normal strength and harmonious functioning in all muscles so that you use all your muscles equally with greater ease and flexibility. With all the muscles being balanced and strengthened they are no longer working against each other thereby eliminating your pain. Fascia tightness and inflammation are also healed. None of these problems require any surgical treatment and surgery was never an effective option.

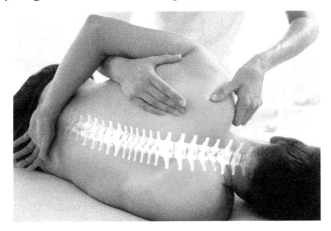

Stretching tight, inflamed muscles and fascia

The same is true for all muscle pain management interventions. All of these pain problems are due to musculoskeletal imbalance. Surgery will only serve to make the problem worse and then you will still need the stretching/strengthening therapy that you needed to do in the first place. Surgery only adds to the problem to make it worse, as there was nothing to "fix" in the first place. Surgery will not restore strength and balance. Surgery is also irreversible. Pain management therapy is only treating the symptoms (maybe) and not addressing the specific cause. Unnecessary spinal injections, nerve ablation and narcotic usage can be avoided.

"All truths are easy to understand once discovered."

—Galileo

As for neck, upper back, and shoulder pain, the same imbalance mechanisms occur. The shoulder girdles are the main structures for support of the upper body and posture. Most of the upper body and neck muscles attach in some way to the shoulder girdles. Weakness or imbalance in any of the shoulder girdle muscles can lead to weakness, spasm and pain. The shoulder girdle is the most complicated joint in the body because of the vast range of motion it is capable of moving through. This complex movement is made possible by the numerous muscles attached to it that make up the shoulder girdle on both sides. When you add having to balance your head on your neck and shoulders, you have a perfect set up for neck and upper back pain. The neck muscles are constantly working to support the head (which typically weighs about 10-11 pounds) and shoulders. The only time they can ever rest is when you are laying down.

Neck, upper back and shoulder pain all comes down to muscle imbalance and loss of flexibility. Neck and head pain frequently go together. Patients may have persistent headaches that no doctor seems to be able to obtain lasting relief. Many of these patients actually have inflammation in their upper neck (occipital neuralgia) and lower neck muscles (cervicalgia), causing their headaches and neck pain. This inflammation leads to fascia irritation, muscle spasm, pain and continued headaches. This inflammation is another physical finding that will not show up on MRI scanning. Diagnosis is made by careful, hands on examination and feeling the muscles of the neck and back. Treatment of all the inflammation frequently will resolve the neck and head pain. Self-administered exercise, stretching and massage are all beneficial. A unique and effective way to apply self-massage is with the use of a "muscle massage gun." This device allows you to apply deep, directed massage therapy to sore, tight muscles.

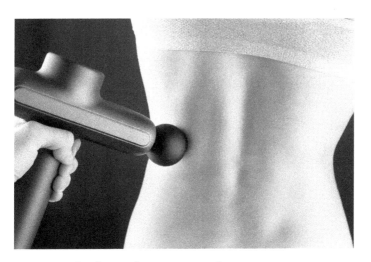

Back muscle massage with massage gun

Upper back and shoulder pain can be a direct result of weak muscles having to compensate for by other upper body muscles. This results in a forward head posture, which then rounds off your shoulders. To your neck muscles, your head now feels five pounds heavier and the neck muscles have to work even harder to pull the head up. Have you ever noticed someone or even yourself having uneven shoulders, with one higher than the other? Or others with their shoulder rolled forward, causing a slumped posture. People will be telling you to "stand up straight" all the time. This is a classic finding in upper body muscle weakness and imbalance.

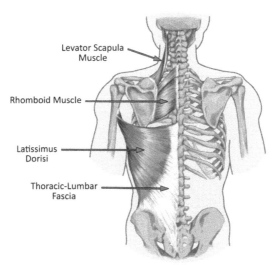

Commonly strained fascia and neck/back muscles

The levator scapula, trapezius and rhomboid muscles are all bad actors when it comes to upper back and neck pain. Trapezius strain and spasm cause upper back and neck pain. Levator scapula strain causes lateral neck pain and occipital headaches. Rhomboid strain is particularly painful in that it can cause severe pain under the shoulder blade as well as mid-upper back. Rhomboid strain needs a therapist for treatment, as you cannot easily do this yourself.

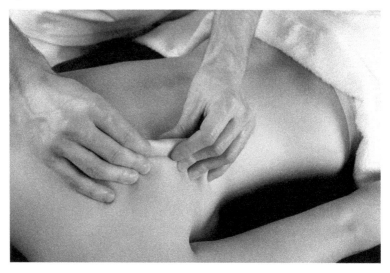

Manual stretching of rhomboid muscle and fascia

The other problem with stooped posture is that it tilts your head forward and your neck muscles need to work overtime to pull your head up. Long term effects of this are increased lower and upper back pain. People who suffer from head, neck, upper back and shoulder pains are often those with poor posture. Careful examination of these individuals shows spasm of certain muscle groups that attach to the shoulder girdle, upper back and neck. Other muscles of the shoulder girdle are weak, shortened and atrophied. This then creates the same type of pain-spasm cycle, just like the lower back.

"You cannot escape the responsibility of tomorrow by evading it today."

—Abraham Lincoln

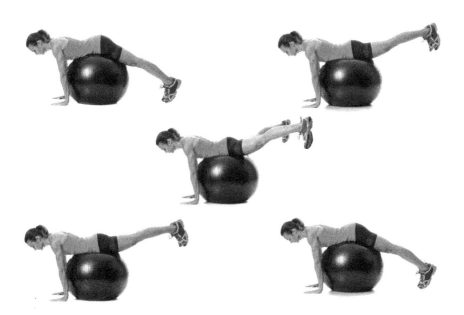

Using yoga ball for back stretching and strengthening

Treating symptoms of pain with massage or generic physical therapy are only temporary. You are only treating the symptoms and not the cause. Routine physical therapy (patients sometimes refer to as "shake and bake") is palliative and temporary at best. Have you ever had physical therapy or massage therapy where you only felt good at the time of the treatment? The next day, you are right back to have the same pain again. That is because the muscle imbalance was not diagnosed nor treated. The only treatment for these muscle imbalances is corrective, hands-on therapy to "reset" the muscles.

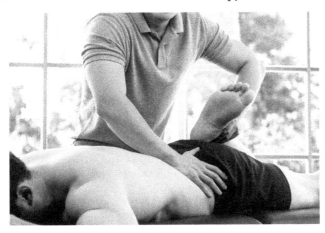

Stretching of the quadriceps muscle

Your therapist, with specialty training in Active Isolated Stretching and Strengthening (AIS), first needs to identify both the weak and overused muscles. Common sense tells us that if you cannot first identify the problem, you cannot fix it. The tight, overused muscles will need to be actively stretched and lengthened to create a balance, followed by strengthening of the weaker muscles to restore the normal, physiological functioning in the neck, upper back, and shoulder girdles.

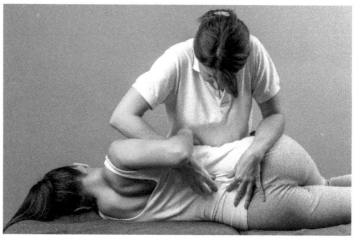

Manual therapy of the thoracic-lumbar muscles and fascia

It is only after these muscles have been lengthened and strengthened is normal function and harmony restored. You will need to continue on your own home stretching and strengthening program to maintain normal muscle flexibility and tone. You need flexibility and strength to maintain a pain-free lifestyle.

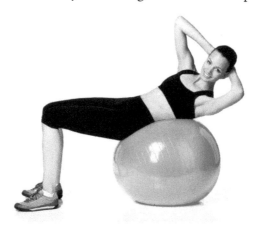

Yoga ball used for muscle stretching and core strengthening

This specifically refers to hands-on, manual physical and exercise therapy. General physical therapy consisting of electrical stimulation, hot packs and ultrasound have not been proven to be effective for healing strained, weak or inflamed soft tissue. Medical fitness conditioning is the specific therapy needed to relieve pain and improve functioning. There are biomechanical laws of the body that explain why pain develops and the necessary steps to correct the problems. This is an area of medicine known as **kinesiology**.[131] Following the biomechanical laws of spinal functioning puts you on the correct road to recovery and a pain free life. Quality-of-life entirely depends on following these biomechanical principles and self-exercise program.

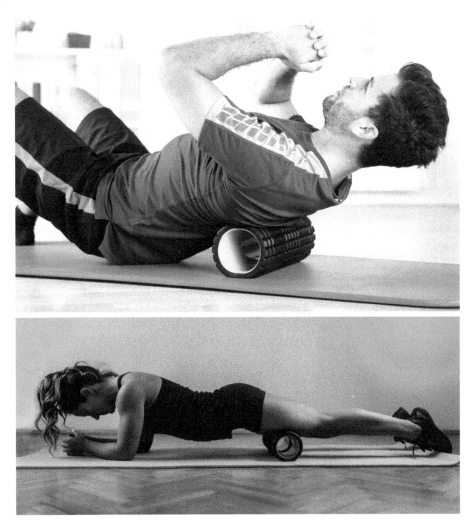

Using foam roller to stretch back and leg muscles

For medication therapy, some studies have shown that acetaminophen, anti-inflammatory agents (such as aspirin, ibuprofen and naproxen) and muscle relaxants may provide some relief in the management of acute or subacute pain.[132],[133],[134] The use of oral steroids has not been shown to be an effective treatment in management of back, neck or leg pain. Studies of back and leg pain with steroid dose packs or longer oral steroid treatment have shown no beneficial effects and expose you to additional complications of this type of therapy.[135] Complications can include increased infections, insomnia, gastritis, increased appetite, weight gain, elevated blood sugar, anxiety and bone fractures. Although rare, avascular necrosis can be a complication of oral steroid use. This condition is characterized by bone death. It is more commonly seen in the hip joints and may need hip joint replacement as the definitive treatment. There is no scientific evidence that oral steroids are effective treatment for neck, back or leg pain. You should never take oral steroids as a treatment for any of these conditions.[136]

For those patients that are considering epidural steroid spine injections or for those with back pain after spine surgery, Platelet Rich Plasma therapy (PRP therapy) is a simple, in-office procedure that can provide natural healing and back pain relief. PRP therapy does not require anesthesia, rehabilitation or any down time. PRP treatment also does not expose the patient to the significant risks associated with epidural steroids. There are numerous published studies showing that epidural steroids are not effective for long-term pain relief.[137,138,139,140,141]

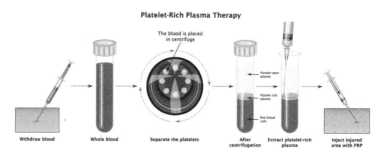

Platelet Rich Plasma therapy (FDA-approved) is derived directly from your own blood. Your blood is drawn in the office and put into a platelet concentrator centrifuge. The platelet rich plasma is drawn off and the rest of the blood is discarded. PRP is a high concentration of your own platelets— the healing component of blood. Contained within platelets are the active healing proteins and growth factors that promote new tissue regeneration and repair damaged tissues.[142]

PRP Therapy is Not Stem Cell Therapy

Growth factors are necessary to initiate tissue healing and regeneration. The PRP is injected into the area that needs healing and tissue regeneration. With concentrated amounts of these regenerative, healing proteins working in an injured area, healing and tissue repair begins. Stem cells, responding to the growth factors, migrate into the area, further aiding in healing. Your body's own healing mechanism generates new, healthy tissue.

Healing can occur in various tissues including tendons, ligaments, muscle and bone. Stem cells can change into whatever tissue type is needed. Along with tissue repair, the regeneration process also stimulates new blood vessel growth to promote the healing process. **Stem cell therapy is not FDA approved for joint and muscle problems.** Stem cells have not been shown to effective at healing damaged tissues. It is also five to six times more expensive than PRP therapy. Stem cell therapy with added PRP can cost nearly ten thousand dollars as some doctors combine stem cells with PRP, claiming benefit, but it is just the PRP that is doing the work.

[From the FDA: Stem cells have not been approved for the treatment of any orthopedic condition, such as osteoarthritis, tendonitis, disc disease, tennis elbow, back pain, hip pain, knee pain, neck pain, or shoulder pain.]

> PRP therapy can often help avoid surgery, or,
> it can help eliminate pain after surgery.

What Issues Does PRP Therapy Treat?

To hear a first-person account from a patient about her experience with PRP, please check out http://sarasotaneurology.com/backpain. PRP therapy is available for treatment of leg pain (sciatica), various neck and back pain conditions and for those afflicted with post-surgical neck or back pain. PRP can work exceptionally well to help heal knee or shoulder pain problems without resorting to surgical treatment. Problems such as torn meniscus or rotator cuff injuries. PRP therapy can be beneficial either before surgery (preferably) or in a post-surgical setting where residual pain is still a problem.

Platelet rich plasma therapy is one of the most effective treatments for a painful foot condition known as plantar fasciitis. PRP has the ability to heal patients that have failed numerous other therapies – both for plantar fasciitis as well as failed back syndrome. It is vastly more effective and safer than any type of epidural steroid procedure. Since PRP is made of your own blood, the healing is safe, effective and entirely natural.

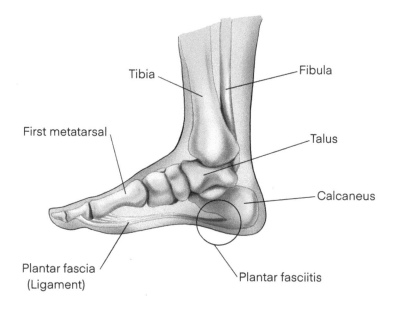

Inflamed plantar fascia causing severe foot pain

What I Want You To Take Away From This Book

Now you know that your neck or back pain is almost never a surgery-requiring problem. You have a choice in making the right decision about the approach you will take to treating your pain. See a back pain specialist who is not a surgeon or pain management specialist, such as an osteopathic physician, neurologist specializing in neck/back pain or physiatrist. Find a therapist trained in kinesiology . Conservative treatment is the recognized protocol for treating almost every case of neck or back pain.

Despite what you may be told, your pain is almost certainly **not** coming from the spine, a bulging disc, or a "pinched nerve," but rather tight, inflamed muscles, tendons, and fascia. MRI findings are misleading, at best. Remember, an MRI is only a picture of your spine. Most spinal abnormalities are very common and have nothing to do with your pain.

Natural healing by the body in combination with hands-on therapy, home exercises, and regular stretching will effectively treat and prevent most cases of neck and back pain. Even non-narcotic medications are an option, but not necessary for complete recovery. Simple over-the-counter analgesics may help temporarily relieve the pain, but are not the solution. Narcotics and oral steroids have no effect on the final resolution of your pain.

AVOID THESE FOUR MISTAKES

1. Do not *first* see a spine surgeon or pain management specialist for your neck or back pain.

2. An MRI is not the first thing you need to find effective treatment for your pain. MRI scanning is commonly never needed.

3. Do not take narcotic pain medications.

4. Do not believe that spine surgery can "fix" your neck or back pain—no matter what is promised to you.

Take care of your body. It's the only place you have to live."

—Jim Rohn

5 THINGS TO START DOING TODAY TO RELIEVE YOUR BACK PAIN

1. Use an ice pack on your back or neck three times daily, for about 10 minutes each session. A reusable soft, gel-type freezer pack is best.

2. Make a copy of the stretching exercises contained in this book and allow time for these every day. Doing these regularly will help prevent future episodes of neck or back pain.

3. For temporary relief, take simple analgesics which are not prescription medications.

4. See a physician who has a conservative (non-surgical) approach to treatment of neck and back pain.

5. Seek out a qualified, hand-on physical therapist, advanced-trained neuromuscular therapist, or acupuncturist for additional treatment.

Start Now, Not Later

Do not put off getting help to relieve your pain and **improve your quality of life**. Take your health into your own hands and do not be led down the primrose path to self-destruction of surgery, narcotics, and ineffective pain management procedures. You can be free of pain with the steps outlined in the book. Start now.

APPENDIX

National Guidelines for Treatment of Cervical, Thoracic and Lumbar Injuries & Pain

Agency for Healthcare Research and Quality – **AHRQ**
U.S. Department of Heath & Human Services
(AHRQ Guidelines Summary NGC-8890 and NGC-9327)

For Acute Cervical, Thoracic, Lumbar Pain:

RECOMMENDED	NOT RECOMMENDED
Non-steroidal anti-inflammatory drugs	Bed rest
Acetaminophen with or without radicular symptoms, for those with contraindications for NSAIDs	Routine use of opioids
Muscle relaxants as a second-line treatment in pain not adequately controlled by NSAIDs	Steroids of any kind
Manual physical therapy with massage for relief of cervical/lumbar pain with an active treatment program focusing on active exercises	Lumbar supports or elastic braces
Limited use of opioids for severe acute cervical or lumbar pain without radicular symptoms	Epidural steroid or facet injections
Self-applications of ice packs to affected areas	Radio frequency nerve ablation
	Spinal surgery or Pain Management

For Subacute Cervical, Thoracic, Lumbar Pain:

RECOMMENDED	NOT RECOMMENDED
Specific stretching and strengthening exercises	Bed rest or traction
Acetaminophen or NSAID therapy	Routine use of opioids
Manual physical therapy with massage for cervical or lumbar pain with active strengthening exercises	Steroids of any kind
Work conditioning or hardening program	Radio frequency nerve ablation
Very limited use of opioids for persistent **severe** cervical or lumbar pain	Epidural steroid or facet injections
Self-application of ice packs or heat to affected areas	Spinal surgery of any type without clear symptoms and objective findings of radiculopathy

AHRQ guidelines are based on the consensus summary of currently published literature.

ABOUT THE AUTHOR

Dr. Kassicieh has been practicing neurology since 1987. He has extensive clinical and research experience in the treatment of head, neck and back pain. With his osteopathic training, Dr. Kassicieh is able to diagnose neck and back problems that involve the muscles, tendons and ligaments. This knowledge also helps in diagnosing spinal problems, or better yet, what is *not* a spinal problem.

In addition to his clinical research experience in treatment of migraine and other headache disorders, he has also been the principle investigator in studies involving treatment of pain—including neck and back pain. These studies involved the non-surgical, non-narcotic treatment of neck and back pain.

Daniel Kassicieh, D.O. FAAN is a dual board-certified osteopathic neurologist. He went to Osteopathic medical school at Kirksville College of Osteopathic Medicine, the first Osteopathic medical school. He then did his neurology training at Ohio State University.

Each year, Dr. Kassicieh travels to impoverished countries to do medical mission work through the organization Hearts Afire.

In his Sarasota, Florida, practice, he is dedicated to helping each person improve the quality of their life. In every case possible, he counsels people how to get healthier and eliminate pain through conservative treatments, avoiding narcotics or falling victim to a spine surgeon's knife. He is renown for providing solutions to headaches, neck, and back pain when no attempts at solving the problem have been successful before.

Connect with Dr. Kassicieh: SarasotaNeurology.com

Medical Missions Service

For over a decade, Dr. Kassicieh has worked with the medical mission charitable organization, Hearts Afire. Hearts Afire is dedicated to provide medical services, food, wells, churches and clinics worldwide to underserviced, impoverished areas. HAF has provided care to people all around the world, including India, Haiti, Dominican Republic and Kenya. Dr. Kassicieh has been on many of these medical mission trips providing medical care and comfort to thousands of people who may never have the opportunity to see a doctor otherwise. He is most recently involved in the HAF Kenya project, over the past 3 years and ongoing. In 2020, HAF built a state-of-the-art hospital-clinic in Eldoret, Kenya, to provide care for over 10 million underserved people. This hospital, is certified in providing maternal care as well as a labor-delivery surgical suite. (Sarasotaneurology.com/medical-missions)

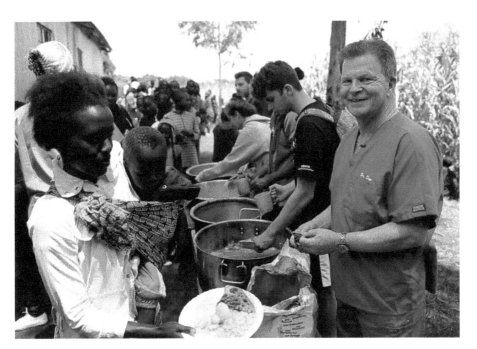

HEARTS AFIRE not only gives medical care to the local population in remote areas, but also provides them with nutritious meals. Above: Mission team, Baharini, Africa

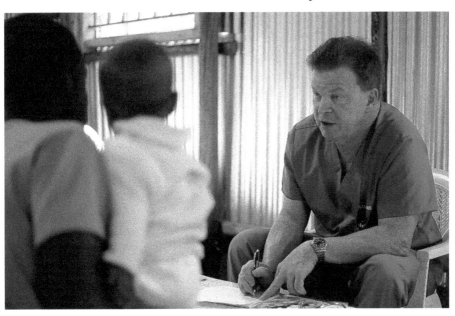

Dr. Kassicieh, providing medical care to men, women, children, and babies as part of his medical mission work with HEARTS AFIRE (Baharini, Africa)

ACKNOWLEDGMENTS

I would like to express my thanks and gratitude to all those who have made this book possible. First, my publisher, Barbara Dee. Without her encouragement and help, I could not have completed this project. Her team at Suncoast Digital Press provided high-level expertise, including the creation of many of the images I wanted to use as a help to readers. Secondly, my IT/video/graphics guru, Bob Stoughton. Bob is truly a graphics pro. His wizardry was invaluable in illustrating this book. Thanks to my office manager, Darla, who kept telling me, "You have to get that book done, Doc." My deepest appreciation to the many that supported me directly and indirectly, with their words of support to keep me going. My special thanks and gratitude to my father, an osteopathic physician, who taught me the fine art of hands-on diagnosis and treatment; to Dr. Harvey Kaltsas, acupuncture physician extraordinaire, whose knowledge in this field was invaluable; and to Terry Simes, Olympic trainer whose skills and knowledge of kinesiology have helped me with this book and many grateful patients. Lastly, I am grateful for the Internet, which has made research fast and much easier.

REFERENCES

1   Carragee EJ. Clinical practice. Persistent low back pain. *N Engl J Med.* 2005 May 5;352(18):1891-8.

2   Jarvik JG, Deyo RA. Diagnostic evaluation of low back pain with emphasis on imaging. *Ann Intern Med.* 2002 Oct 1;137(7):586-97.

3   Lateef H, Patel D. What is the role of imaging in acute low back pain?. *Curr Rev Musculoskelet Med.* 2009;2(2):69-73.

4   Carette S, Leclaire R, Marcoux S, Morin F, Blaise GA, St-Pierre A, Truchon R, Parent F, Levésque J, Bergeron V, Montminy P, Blanchette C. Epidural corticosteroid injections for sciatica due to herniated nucleus pulposus. *N Engl J Med.* 1997 Jun 5;336(23):1634-40.

5   Malanga GA, Cruz Colon EJ. Myofascial low back pain: a review. *Phys Med Rehabil Clin N Am.* 2010 Nov;21(4):711-24.

6   Ibid

7   Lateef H, Patel D. What is the role of imaging in acute low back pain?. *Curr Rev Musculoskelet Med.* 2009;2(2):69-73.

8   Licciardone, J.C., Brimhall, A.K. & King, L.N. Osteopathic manipulative treatment for low back pain: a systematic review and meta-analysis of randomized controlled trials. *BMC Musculoskelet Disord 6*, 43 (2005).

9   Trampisch HJ, Molsberger A. German Acupuncture Trials (GERAC) for chronic low back pain: randomized, multicenter, blinded, parallel-group trial with 3 groups. *Arch Intern Med.* 2007 Sep 24;167(17):1892-8.

10 Preyde M. Effectiveness of massage therapy for subacute low-back pain: a randomized controlled trial. *CMAJ.* 2000 Jun 27;162(13):1815-20.

11 Cherkin DC, Eisenberg D, Sherman KJ, Barlow W, Kaptchuk TJ, Street J, Deyo RA. Randomized trial comparing traditional Chinese medical acupuncture, therapeutic massage, and self-care education for chronic low back pain. *Arch Intern Med.* 2001 Apr 23;161(8):1081-8.

12 Pope MH, Phillips RB, Haugh LD, Hsieh CY, MacDonald L, Haldeman S. A prospective randomized three-week trial of spinal manipulation, transcutaneous muscle stimulation, massage and corset in the treatment of subacute low back pain. *Spine* (Phila Pa 1976). 1994 Nov 15;19(22):2571-7.

13 Cherkin DC, Sherman KJ, Kahn J, Wellman R, Cook AJ, Johnson E, Erro J, Delaney K, Deyo RA. A comparison of the effects of 2 types of massage and usual care on chronic low back pain: a randomized, controlled trial. *Ann Intern Med.* 2011 Jul 5;155(1):1-9.

14 Qaseem A, Wilt TJ, McLean RM, Forciea MA; Clinical Guidelines Committee of the American College of Physicians. Noninvasive Treatments for Acute, Subacute, and Chronic Low Back Pain: A Clinical Practice Guideline From the American College of Physicians. *Ann Intern Med.* 2017 Apr 4;166(7):514-530.

15 Ibid

16 Turner JA, Avins AL, James K, Wald JT, Kallmes DF, Jarvik JG. Systematic literature review of imaging features of spinal degeneration in asymptomatic populations. *AJNR Am J Neuroradiol.* 2015 Apr;36(4):811-6.

17 Okada E, Matsumoto M, Fujiwara H, Toyama Y. Disc degeneration of cervical spine on MRI in patients with lumbar disc herniation: comparison study with asymptomatic volunteers. *Eur Spine J.* 2011 Apr;20(4):585-91.

18 Jensen MC, Kelly AP, Brant-Zawadzki MN. MRI of degenerative disease of the lumbar spine. *Magn Reson Q.* 1994 Sep;10(3):173-90.

19 Waris E, Eskelin M, Hermunen H, Kiviluoto O, Paajanen H. Disc degeneration in low back pain: a 17-year follow-up study using magnetic resonance imaging. *Spine* (Phila Pa 1976). 2007 Mar 15;32(6):681-4.

20 Turner JA, Avins AL, James K, Wald JT, Kallmes DF, Jarvik JG. Systematic literature review of imaging features of spinal degeneration in asymptomatic populations. *AJNR Am J Neuroradiol.* 2015 Apr;36(4):811-6.

21 Waldman P, Armstrong D. Doctors Getting Rich With Fusion Surgery Debunked by Studies. Bloomberg News. 2010 Dec 30.

22 Brouwer PA, Brand R, van den Akker-van Marle ME, et al. Percutaneous laser disc decompression versus conventional microdiscectomy for patients with sciatica: Two-year results of a randomised controlled trial. *Interv Neuroradiol.* 2017;23(3):313-324.

23   Sinicropi S. 5 Reasons Why Spine Surgery Will Boom in the Next Decade. *Becker's Spine Review*, March 2017, Vol 2017 No. 2.

24   Mitchell NS, Catenacci VA, Wyatt HR, Hill JO. Obesity: overview of an epidemic. *Psychiatr Clin North Am*. 2011;34(4):717-732.

25   Milby A. Failed Back Surgery Syndrome: When the Pain Comes Back After Surgery. Penn Med Neuroscience Blog, 2018 Sept 05.

26   Spoor AB, Öner FC. Minimally invasive spine surgery in chronic low back pain patients. *J Neurosurg Sci*. 2013;57(3):203-218.

27   Chou R. Low back pain (chronic). *BMJ Clin Evid*. 2010 Oct 8;2010:1116.

28   Spoor AB, Öner FC. Minimally invasive spine surgery in chronic low back pain patients. *J Neurosurg Sci*. 2013 Sep;57(3):203-18.

29   Chou R, Qaseem A, Snow V, Casey D, Cross JT Jr, Shekelle P, Owens DK; Clinical Efficacy Assessment Subcommittee of the American College of Physicians; American College of Physicians; American Pain Society Low Back Pain Guidelines Panel. Diagnosis and treatment of low back pain: a joint clinical practice guideline from the American College of Physicians and the American Pain Society. *Ann Intern Med*. 2007 Oct 2;147(7):478-91.

30   Atlas SJ, Deyo RA. Evaluating and managing acute low back pain in the primary care setting. *J Gen Intern Med*. 2001 Feb;16(2):120-31.

31   Andersson GBJ. *The Epidemiology of Spinal Disorders*. In: Frymoyer JW, Ducker TB, Hadler NM, Kostuik JP, Weinstein JN, Whitecloud TS, editors. *The Adult Spine: Principles and Practice*.Philadelphia, PA: Lippincott-Raven; 1997. pp. 93–141.

32   Derek J. Emery, MD, FRCPC; Kaveh G. Shojania, MD, FRCPC; Alan J. Forster, MD, FRCPC; et al. Overuse of Magnetic Resonance Imaging. *JAMA Intern Med*. 2013;173(9):823-825.

33   Chou R, Deyo RA, Jarvik JG. Appropriate use of lumbar imaging for evaluation of low back pain. *Radiol Clin North Am*. 2012 Jul;50(4):569-85.

34   Chou R, Qaseem A, Owens DK, Shekelle P; Clinical Guidelines Committee of the American College of Physicians. Diagnostic imaging for low back pain: advice for high-value health care from the American College of Physicians. *Ann Intern Med*. 2011 Feb 1;154(3):181-9.

35   Practice parameters: magnetic resonance imaging in the evaluation of low back syndrome (summary statement). Report of the Quality Standards Subcommittee of the American Academy of Neurology. *Neurology*. 1994 Apr;44(4):767-70.

36   Kallmes DF, Jarvik JG. Systematic literature review of imaging features of spinal degeneration in asymptomatic populations. *AJNR Am J Neuroradiol.* 2015 Apr;36(4):811-6.

37   Gabrielle Hultman (1994) Back-healthy men, 45–55 years old, their characteristics and environment compared to men with intermittent and chronic low back pain a cross-sectional study, *Acta Orthopaedica Scandinavica*, 65:sup256, 116-116.

38   Duthey, B PhD, WHO Background Paper 6.24, Low back pain, March 2013.

39   Chiu CC, Chuang TY, Chang KH, Wu CH, Lin PW, Hsu WY. The probability of spontaneous regression of lumbar herniated disc: a systematic review. *Clin Rehabil.* 2015 Feb;29(2):184-95.

40   Brinjikji W, Luetmer PH, Comstock B, Bresnahan BW, et al. Systematic literature review of imaging features of spinal degeneration in asymptomatic populations. *AJNR Am J Neuroradiol.* 2015 Apr;36(4):811-6.

41   Friedly JL, Comstock BA, Turner JA et al (2014) A randomized trial of epidural glucocorticoid injections for spinal stenosis. *N Engl J Med* 371:11–21

42   Shaughnessy AF. Epidural Steroid Not Better Than Placebo Injection for Sciatica and Spinal Stenosis Pain and Function. *Am Fam Physician.* 2016 Feb 15;93(4):315-6.

43   Carette S, M.D., Leclaire R, M.D., Marcoux S, M.D., et al. Epidural Corticosteroid Injections for Sciatica Due to Herniated Nucleus Pulposus. *N Engl J Med* 1997; 336:1634-1640.

44   Hildebrandt J. [Relevance of nerve blocks in treating and diagnosing low back pain--is the quality decisive?]. Schmerz. 2001;15(6):474-483.

45   Staal JB, de Bie RA, de Vet HC, Hildebrandt J, Nelemans P. Injection therapy for subacute and chronic low back pain: an updated Cochrane review. *Spine* (Phila Pa 1976). 2009 Jan 1;34(1):49-59.

46   hopkinsmedicine.org/health/conditions-and-diseases/epidural-corticosteroid-injections

47   Shim, JH. Limitations of spinal cord stimulation for pain management, *Korean J Anesthesiol.* 2015 Aug; 68(4): 321–322.

48   Turner JA, Hollingworth W, Comstock BA, Deyo RA. Spinal cord stimulation for failed back surgery syndrome: outcomes in a workers' compensation setting. *Pain.* 2010 Jan;148(1):14-25.

49   Chou R, Huffman LH; American Pain Society; American College of
      Physicians. Nonpharmacologic therapies for acute and chronic low back
      pain: a review of the evidence for an American Pain Society/American
      College of Physicians clinical practice guideline. *Ann Intern Med.* 2007
      Oct 2;147(7):492-504.

50   Gautschi OP, Hildebrandt G, Cadosch D. Acute low back pain-
      -assessment and management. *Praxis* (Bern 1994). 2008 Jan
      23;97(2):58-68.

51   Kinkade S. Evaluation and treatment of acute low back pain.
      Am Fam Physician. 2007 Apr 15;75(8):1181-8.

52   Neeland IJ, Ross R, Després JP, et al; International Atherosclerosis
      Society; International Chair on Cardiometabolic Risk
      Working Group on Visceral Obesity. Visceral and ectopic fat,
      atherosclerosis, and cardiometabolic disease: a position statement.
      Lancet Diabetes Endocrinol. 2019 Sep;7(9):715-725.

53   Moghaddam AA, Woodward M, Huxley R. Obesity and risk of
      colorectal cancer: a meta-analysis of 31 studies with 70,000 events.
      Cancer Epidemiol Biomarkers Prev. 2007 Dec;16(12):2533-47.

54   Misra D, Fielding RA, Felson DT, Niu J, Brown C, Nevitt M, Lewis
      CE, Torner J, Neogi T; MOST study. Risk of Knee Osteoarthritis With
      Obesity, Sarcopenic Obesity, and Sarcopenia. *Arthritis Rheumatol.* 2019
      Feb;71(2):232-237.

55   Donnally III CJ, Butler AJ, Varacallo M. Lumbosacral Disc Injuries.
      [Updated 2020 Jul 19]. In: StatPearls [Internet]. Treasure Island (FL):
      StatPearls Publishing; 2020 Jan-.

56   Lateef, H., Patel, D. What is the role of imaging in acute low back
      pain?. *Curr Rev Musculoskelet Med 2,* 69–73 (2009).

57   Ibid

58   Spoor AB, Öner FC. Minimally invasive spine surgery in chronic low
      back pain patients. *J Neurosurg Sci.* 2013 Sep;57(3):203-18.

59   Brinjikji W, Luetmer PH, Comstock B, et al. Systematic literature
      review of imaging features of spinal degeneration in asymptomatic
      populations. *AJNR Am J Neuroradiol.* 2015 Apr;36(4):811-6.

60   Starfield B. Is US health really the best in the world? *JAMA.* 2000 Jul
      26;284(4):483-5.

61   Kurpad, S. Laser Spine Surgery: What Does the Science Say?. Med.
      College of Wisconsin. 2018; Mar 8.

62   Deyo RA, Bass JE. Lifestyle and low-back pain. The influence of smoking and obesity. Spine (Phila Pa 1976). 1989 May;14(5):501-6. Stern, J, Lasers in Spine Surgery: A Review. *Spineline.* 2019; Sept-Oct: 17-20.

63   Sandén B, Försth P, Michaëlsson K. Smokers show less improvement than nonsmokers two years after surgery for lumbar spinal stenosis: a study of 4555 patients from the Swedish spine register. *Spine* (Phila Pa 1976). 2011 Jun;36(13):1059-64.

64   Berman D, Oren JH, Bendo J, Spivak J. The Effect of Smoking on Spinal Fusion. *Int J Spine Surg.* 2017 Nov 28;11(4):29.

65   Sandén B, Försth P, Michaëlsson K. Smokers show less improvement than nonsmokers two years after surgery for lumbar spinal stenosis: a study of 4555 patients from the Swedish spine register. *Spine* (Phila Pa 1976). 2011 Jun;36(13):1059-64.

66   Epstein NE. Should anyone perform percutaneous endoscopic laser diskectomy and percutaneous lumbar disc decompressions? *Surg Neurol Int.* 2016 Dec 26;7(Suppl 42):S1080-S1084.

67   Substance Abuse and Mental Health Services Administration. Drug Abuse Warning Network: selected tables of national estimates of drug-related emergency department visits. Rockville, MD: Center for Behavioral Health Statistics and Quality, SAMHSA; 2010.

68   Hah J, Hernandez-Boussard T. Defining Postoperative Opioid Needs Among Preoperative Opioid Users. *JAMA Surg.* 2018 Jul 1;153(7):689-690.

69   Ibid

70   Krebs EE, Gravely A, Nugent S, Jensen AC, DeRonne B, Goldsmith ES, Kroenke K, Bair MJ, Noorbaloochi S. Effect of Opioid vs Nonopioid Medications on Pain-Related Function in Patients With Chronic Back Pain or Hip or Knee Osteoarthritis Pain: The SPACE Randomized Clinical Trial. *JAMA.* 2018 Mar 6;319(9):872-882.

71   Shim H, Rose J, Halle S, Shekane P. Complex regional pain syndrome: a narrative review for the practicing clinician. *Br J Anaesth.* 2019 Aug;123(2):e424-e433.

72   Burton CV. Failed back surgery patients: the alarm bells are ringing. *Surg Neurol.* 2006 Jan;65(1):5-6.

73   Sinicropi S. 5 Reasons Why Spine Surgery Will Boom in the Next Decade. *Becker's Spine Review*, March 2017, Vol 2017 No. 2.

74   Ibid

75   Deyo RA, Gray DT, Kreuter W, Mirza S, Martin BI. United States trends in lumbar fusion surgery for degenerative conditions. *Spine* (Phila Pa 1976). 2005 Jun 15;30(12):1441-5; discussion 1446-7.

76   Weinstein JN, Lurie JD, Olson PR, Bronner KK, Fisher ES. United States' trends and regional variations in lumbar spine surgery: 1992-2003. *Spine* (Phila Pa 1976). 2006 Nov 1;31(23):2707-14.

77   Deyo RA, Mirza SK. The case for restraint in spinal surgery: does quality management have a role to play? *Eur Spine J* (2009) 18 (Suppl 3):S331–S337.

78   Freburger JK, Holmes GM, Agans RP, Jackman AM, Darter JD, Wallace AS, Castel LD, Kalsbeek WD, Carey TS. The rising prevalence of chronic low back pain. *Arch Intern Med*. 2009 Feb 9;169(3):251-8.

79   Ibid

80   Ibid

81   Ibid

82   Krebs EE, Gravely A, Nugent S, et al. Effect of Opioid vs Nonopioid Medications on Pain-Related Function in Patients With Chronic Back Pain or Hip or Knee Osteoarthritis Pain: The SPACE Randomized Clinical Trial. *JAMA*. 2018;319(9):872–882.

83   Mafi JN, McCarthy EP, Davis RB, Landon BE. Worsening trends in the management and treatment of back pain. *JAMA Intern Med*. 2013 Sep 23;173(17):1573-81.

84   Wilson N, Kariisa M, Seth P, Smith H IV, Davis NL. Drug and Opioid-Involved Overdose Deaths—United States, 2017–2018. *MMWR Morb Mortal Wkly Rep* 2020;69:290–297.

85   Mafi JN, McCarthy EP, Davis RB, Landon BE. Worsening trends in the management and treatment of back pain. *JAMA Intern Med*. 2013;173(17):1573-1581.

86   ibid

87   ibid

88   Deyo RA, Mirza SK, Turner JA, Martin BI. Overtreating chronic back pain: time to back off?. *J Am Board Fam Med*. 2009;22(1):62-68.

89   Deyo RA, Smith DH, Johnson ES, et al. Opioids for back pain patients: primary care prescribing patterns and use of services. *J Am Board Fam Med*. 2011;24(6):717-727.

90   ibid

91   Krebs EE, Gravely A, Nugent S, et al. Effect of opioid vs nonopioid medications on pain-related function in patients with chronic back pain or hip or knee osteoarthritis pain: the SPACE randomized clinical trial. *JAMA*. 2018;319(9):872-882.

92   Liuke M, Solovieva S, Lamminen A, Luoma K, Leino-Arjas P, Luukkonen R, Riihimäki H. Disc degeneration of the lumbar spine in relation to overweight. *Int J Obes (Lond)*. 2005 Aug;29(8):903-8.

93   Rush AJ, Polatin P, Gatchel RJ. Depression and chronic low back pain: establishing priorities in treatment. *Spine* (Phila Pa 1976). 2000 Oct 15;25(20):2566-71.

94   Cherkin, Daniel C., PhD; Deyo, Richard A., MD, MPH et. al, An International Comparison of Back Surgery Rates; *Spine*: June 1, 1994, Volume 19, Issue 11, pp. 1201–1206.

95   Deyo RA, Gray DT, Kreuter W, Mirza S, Martin BI. United States trends in lumbar fusion surgery for degenerative conditions. *Spine* (Phila Pa 1976) 2005;30:1441–5.

96   Gaskin DJ, Richard P. The Economic Costs of Pain in the United States. In: Institute of Medicine (US) Committee on Advancing Pain Research, Care, and Education. Relieving Pain in America: A Blueprint for Transforming Prevention, Care, Education, and Research. Washington (DC): National Academies Press (US); 2011. Appendix C.

97   Global Health Estimates 2016: Years Lost Due to Disability 2000-2016, 20 Leading Causes, Geneva, World Health Organization; 2018.

98   Whoriskey P, Keating D. Spinal fusions serve as a case study for debate over when certain surgeries are necessary. Washington Post. October 27, 2013.

99   Turner JA, Ersek M, Herron L, Haselkorn J, Kent D, Ciol MA, Deyo R. Patient outcomes after lumbar spinal fusions. *JAMA*. 1992 Aug 19;268(7):907-11.

100   Dhillon KS. Spinal Fusion for Chronic Low Back Pain: A 'Magic Bullet' or Wishful Thinking?. *Malays Orthop J*. 2016;10(1):61-68.

101   Bigos S, Bowyer O, Braen G. Acute Low Back Problems in Adults. Rockville (MD): Agency for Health Care Policy and Research (AHCPR); 1994 Dec.

102   Whoriskey P, Keating D. Spinal fusions serve as a case study for debate over when certain surgeries are necessary. Washington Post. October 27, 2013.

103   Cherkin, Daniel C., PhD; Deyo, Richard A., MD, MPH et. al, An International Comparison of Back Surgery Rates; *Spine*: June 1, 1994, Volume 19, Issue 11, pp. 1201–1206.

104 Nguyen TH, Randolph DC, et.al., Long-term outcomes of lumbar fusion among workers' compensation subjects: a historical cohort study, *Spine*. 2011 Feb 15;36(4):320-31.

105 ibid

106 Klekamp J, McCarty E, Spengler DM. Results of elective lumbar discectomy for patients involved in the workers' compensation system. *J Spinal Disord*. 1998 Aug;11(4):277-82.

107 Johnson H, Paulozzi L, Porucznik C, Mack K, Herter B. Decline in Drug Overdose Deaths After State Policy Changes—Florida, 2010–2012. *CDC MMWR*. July 4, 2014 / 63(26);569-574.

108 Hedegaard, H M.D., Miniño, AM M.P.H., Warner,M Ph.D Drug Overdose Deaths in the United States 1999–2017, *NCHS Data Brief No. 329*, November 2018.

109 Whoriskey P, Keating D. Spinal fusions serve as a case study for debate over when certain surgeries are necessary. Washington Post. October 27, 2013.

110 Woolston C. Back Surgery, *Healthday*. Dec 31, 2019.

111 Malanga GA, Cruz Colon EJ. Myofascial low back pain: a review. *Phys Med Rehabil Clin N Am*. 2010 Nov;21(4):711-24.

112 Deyo RA, Mirza SK. Trends and variations in the use of spine surgery. *Clin Orthop Relat Res*. 2006 Feb;443:139-46.

113 Forsth P, Olafsson G, Carlsson T, et al. A randomized, controlled trial of fusion surgery for lumbar spinal stenosis. *N. Engl. J. Med.*, 374 (15) (2016), pp. 1413-1423.

114 Skeppholm M, Henriques T, Tullberg T. Higher reoperation rate following cervical disc replacement in a retrospective, long-term comparative study of 715 patients. *Eur Spine J* (2017) 26:2434–2440.

115 Deyo RA, Mirza SK, Turner JA, Martin BI. Overtreating chronic back pain: time to back off?. *J Am Board Fam Med*. 2009;22(1):62-68.

116 Dhillon KS. Spinal Fusion for Chronic Low Back Pain: A 'Magic Bullet' or Wishful Thinking?. *Malays Orthop J*. 2016;10(1):61-68.

117 Bogduk N, Andersson G. Is spinal surgery effective for back pain? *F1000 Med Rep*. 2009 Jul 27;1:60.

118 ibid

119 ibid

120 Dhillon KS. Spinal Fusion for Chronic Low Back Pain: A 'Magic Bullet' or Wishful Thinking?. *Malays Orthop J*. 2016;10(1):61-68.

121   Willems P. Decision making in surgical treatment of chronic low back pain: the performance of prognostic tests to select patients for lumbar spinal fusion. *Acta Orthop Suppl.* 2013 Feb;84(349):1-35.

122   Wright, Michael H.; Denney, Leann C. A Comprehensive Review of Spinal Arachnoiditis, Orthopaedic Nursing: May-June 2003 - Volume 22 - Issue 3 - p 215-219.

123   ibid

124   Daniell JR, Osti OL. Failed Back Surgery Syndrome: A Review Article. *Asian Spine J.* 2018;12(2):372-379.

125   Alf L Nachemson (1993) Evaluation of results in lumbar spine surgery, *ActaOrthopaedica Scandinavica*, 64:sup251, 130-133.

126   Gum JL, Glassman SD, Carreon LY. Is type of compensation a predictor of outcome after lumbar fusion? *Spine* (Phila Pa 1976). 2013 Mar 1;38(5):443-8.

127   Carreon LY, Glassman SD, Kantamneni NR, Mugavin MO, Djurasovic M. Clinical outcomes after posterolateral lumbar fusion in workers' compensation patients: a case-control study. *Spine* (Phila Pa 1976). 2010 Sep 1;35(19):1812-7.

128   Kumar MN, Baklanov A, Chopin D. Correlation between sagittal plane changes and adjacent segment degeneration following lumbar spine fusion. *Eur Spine J.* 2001 Aug;10(4):314-9.

129   Baber Z, Erdek MA. Failed back surgery syndrome: current perspectives. *J Pain Res.* 2016 Nov 7;9:979-987.

130   https://my.clevelandclinic.org/health/diseases/12054-myofascial-pain-syndrome

131   Eardley S, Brien S, Little P, Prescott P, Lewith G. Professional kinesiology practice for chronic low back pain: single-blind, randomised controlled pilot study. *Forsch Komplementmed.* 2013;20(3):180-8.

132   van Tulder MW, Touray T, Furlan AD, Solway S, Bouter LM. Muscle relaxants for non-specific low back pain. Cochrane Database Syst Rev. 2003;2003(2):CD004252.

133   Morelli KM, Brown LB, Warren GL. Effect of NSAIDs on Recovery From Acute Skeletal Muscle Injury: A Systematic Review and Meta-analysis. *Am J Sports Med.* 2018 Jan;46(1):224-233.

134   Chou R, Qaseem A, Snow V, Casey D, Cross JT Jr, Shekelle P, Owens DK; Clinical Efficacy Assessment Subcommittee of the American College of Physicians; American College of Physicians; American Pain Society Low Back Pain Guidelines Panel. Diagnosis and treatment of low back pain: a joint clinical practice guideline from the American College of Physicians and the American Pain Society. *Ann Intern Med.* 2007 Oct 2;147(7):478-91.

135   Johnson MJ, Neher JO, St. Anna L. How effective—and safe— are systemic steroids for acute low back pain? *J Fam Pract.* 2011 May;60(5):297-298.

136   ibid

137   Chou R, Hashimoto R, Friedly J, Fu R, Bougatsos C, Dana T, Sullivan SD, Jarvik J. Epidural Corticosteroid Injections for Radiculopathy and Spinal Stenosis: A Systematic Review and Meta-analysis. *Ann Intern Med.* 2015 Sep 1;163(5):373-81.

138   Choi HJ, Hahn S, Kim CH, Jang BH, Park S, Lee SM, Park JY, Chung CK, Park BJ. Epidural steroid injection therapy for low back pain: a meta-analysis. *Int J Technol Assess Health Care.* 2013 Jul;29(3):244-53.

139   Iversen T, Solberg TK, Romner B, et al. Effect of caudal epidural steroid or saline injection in chronic lumbar radiculopathy: multicentre, blinded, randomised controlled trial. *BMJ.* 2011;343:d5278.

140   Friedly JL, Comstock BA, Turner JA, Heagerty PJ, Deyo RA, Sullivan SD, Bauer Z, Bresnahan BW, Avins AL, Nedeljkovic SS, Nerenz DR, Standaert C, Kessler L, Akuthota V, Annaswamy T, Chen A, Diehn F, Firtch W, Gerges FJ, Gilligan C, Goldberg H, Kennedy DJ, Mandel S, Tyburski M, Sanders W, Sibell D, Smuck M, Wasan A, Won L, Jarvik JG. A randomized trial of epidural glucocorticoid injections for spinal stenosis. *N Engl J Med.* 2014 Jul 3;371(1):11-21.

141   Atlas SJ. Epidural steroid injections are not effective for patients with lumbar spinal stenosis. *Evid Based Med.* 2015 Feb;20(1):16.

142   Dhillon RS, Schwarz EM, Maloney MD. Platelet-rich plasma therapy - future or trend?. *Arthritis Res Ther.* 2012;14(4):219.

CPSIA information can be obtained
at www.ICGtesting.com
Printed in the USA
BVHW020322140721
611909BV00001B/8